D0460824

Artificial Organs

Look for these and other books in the Lucent
Overview series:

Artificial Organs

by Judith Janda Presnall

LUCENT
BOOKS

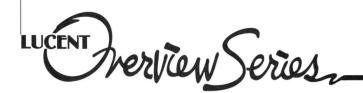

LUCENT Overview Series

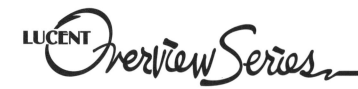

Library of Congress Cataloging-in-Publication Data

Presnall, Judith Janda.
    Artificial organs / by Judith Janda Presnall.
        p.   cm. — (Lucent overview series)
    Includes bibliographical references and index.
    Summary: Examines the history and development of artificial
body parts and their recent improvement through electronic
technology.
    ISBN 1-56006-257-6 (alk. paper)
    1. Artificial organs—Juvenile literature.   [1. Artificial
organs.]   I. Title.   II. Series.
RD130.P74   1996
617.9'5—dc20   95-30529
                                                              CIP
                                                               AC

To Lewis and Alice Presnall

Acknowledgments

The author wishes to express her gratitude to the many people who reviewed manuscript pages and donated their time and efforts in the creation of this book:

Drs. Willem J. Kolff, Richard Normann, George M. Pantalos, Division of Artificial Organs at the University of Utah College of Medicine, Salt Lake City, Utah; Dr. Susan J. Quaal, Department of Veterans Affairs Medical Center, Salt Lake City, Utah; Dr. Harold H. Sears, Motion Control, Salt Lake City, Utah; Dr. William C. DeVries, Louisville, Kentucky; Dr. Robert C. Eberhart, University of Texas Southwestern Medical School, Dallas, Texas; Dr. Richard Grossman, Director of the Burn Center at Sherman Oaks Hospital and Health Center, Sherman Oaks, California; Dr. W. Scott Calvin, Northridge Ophthalmology Associates, Northridge, California; Maggie Holloway, Pediatric Dialysis Program, University of California, Los Angeles, California; Susan Vogel, South Valley Regional Dialysis Center, Inc., Encino, California; Dilys J. Jones, House Ear Institute, Los Angeles, California; and Southern California dialysis patients Joyce Roscel Joaquin, Robert Mandegar, and Edwin Mota.

Contents

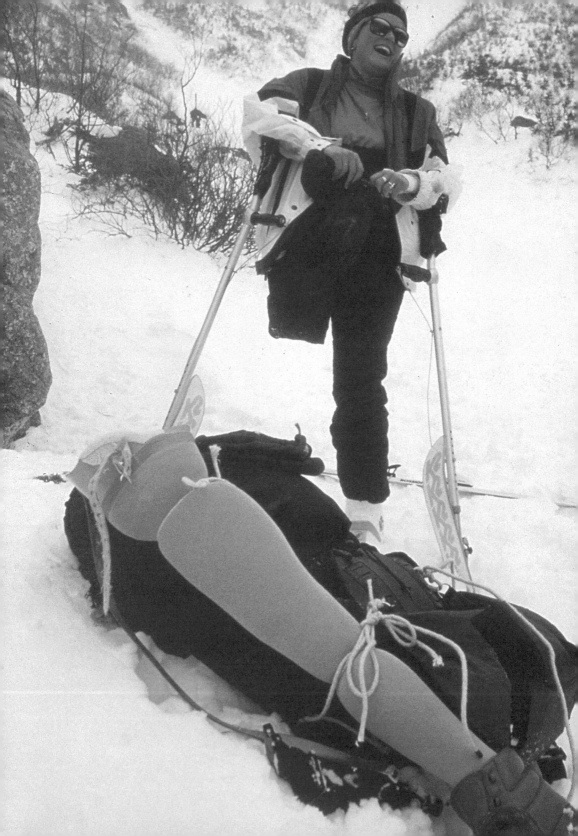

Introduction

THE CHALLENGE OF artificial-organ scientists is to duplicate nature's handiwork by using human technology. Nature can grow a complete person in just nine months. But scientists have taken far longer to develop replacement parts for the human body. However, in recent years scientists have combined an understanding of natural body processes, invention of materials that can be used inside the body, and miniaturization of electronic parts to produce highly sophisticated artificial organs. Bioengineers (those who combine the study of medicine, biology, and engineering) predict that artificial parts will someday be available to replace almost any piece of the human anatomy, except for the brain itself.

In the United States nearly thirteen million procedures that involve artificial organs are performed each year. Artificial organs—sometimes called prostheses—are materials or devices designed either for implantation inside the body or for use outside the body. An artificial organ replaces a faulty or missing part that has been damaged or lost through disease or injury. Sometimes the prosthesis takes over the full-time function of an organ, as with an artificial limb. At other times the human-made part, such as an artificial heart, will be used as a bridge to a transplant. An artificial organ can be permanent, such as arteries and

(Opposite page) After removing her prosthesis, Lisa Niemanis, who lost a leg to cancer, prepares to ski on the slopes of Mount Washington, New Hampshire. Advancements in artificial limb and organ technology have extended and improved the lives of millions of individuals.

9

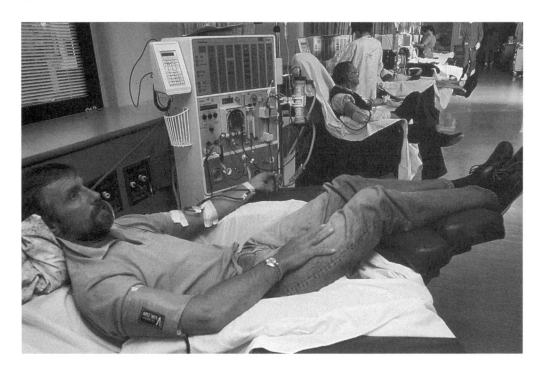

A patient receives computerized hemodialysis on an artificial kidney, a thrice-weekly procedure. The procedure can be done in any dialysis center available worldwide.

heart valves, or it can be temporary, such as a heart-lung machine, which takes over the function of both those organs during open-heart surgery.

The development of artificial organs is crucial because the demand for organ transplants far exceeds available donor organs. Many patients die while awaiting a transplant. In addition, some organs cannot be replaced with donor parts, such as limbs and cochlear hair cells in the ear. Artificial organs give physical mobility and independence to the disabled and allow people to live longer, healthier lives.

For example, before the invention of the artificial kidney in the 1940s, patients with impaired kidneys died when their blood filled with wastes or poisons. Today approximately a half million people survive because of the miracle of the artificial kidney. Also called a dialyzer, the artificial kidney filters wastes from the patient's blood. Because of the hundreds of types of dialyzer machines available worldwide, kidney patients are able to lead normal lives—to go to school, work, and travel.

A more recent invention, the cochlear implant in the inner ear, has restored hearing to many people with no hearing ability. Jane Knight, a young mother who lost her hearing in an accident, told about her experience in the May 1991 issue of *Redbook* magazine. After five silent years a cochlear implant allowed her to hear again. She heard her five-year-old son's voice for the first time. "I love you Mommy," he said. As Knight explains:

> I'm constantly thrilled by everyday sounds. I can hear popcorn popping in the microwave, our dog Rascal snoring and even soft sounds like the hum of the refrigerator, the "shhh" of rain or running water, or my son's tiny feet walking down the hallway.

Incredible success has been achieved in the field of artificial organs since its early beginnings, when strapping a tree branch to the stump of a leg was the only way to replace the missing limb. Modern technology and inventions have led to body implants of arteries and valves, to electronic limbs, and to the modern miracles of electrode brain implants. None of these inventions is the work of one person. They are a result of the combined efforts of medical doctors, engineers, chemists, computer and electronic specialists, and technicians. Working together, these scientists have extended and improved human lives. As research continues, artificial organs promise to be among the most important technologies of the future.

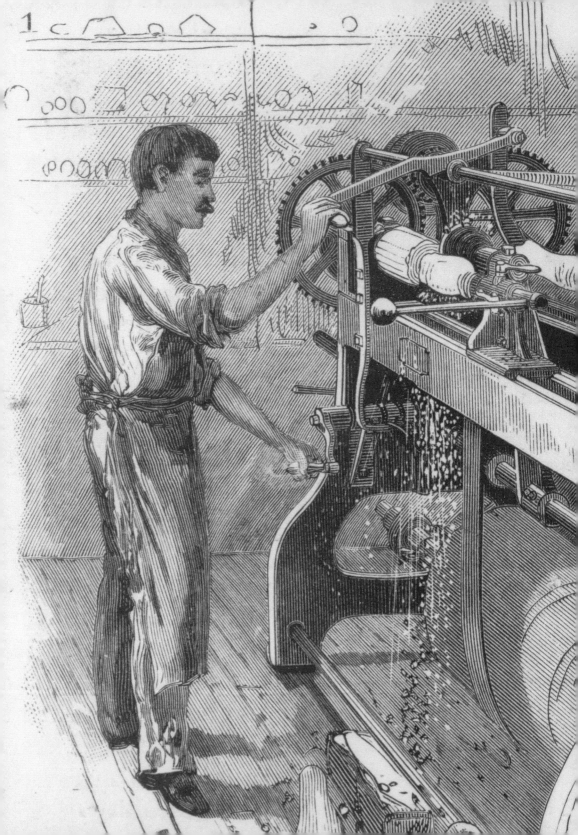

1

Body Parts: From Crude to Functional

THE EARLIEST ARTIFICIAL organs were mostly artificial limbs. They served as crude replacements for faulty or missing arms and legs. From primitive times until the fifteenth century, artificial limbs were made from tree parts. Rough branches were either whittled and attached to amputated leg stumps or used for crutches. These crude parts could perform some basic functions, though nothing approaching the maneuvering ability of a working hand or foot. They did not look like real legs, arms, and hands, either. Nevertheless, these earliest artificial limbs were the beginning of the artificial-organ technology that would emerge over the next few centuries.

Movable joints

The sixteenth century brought about the addition of levers, strings, belts, springs, and joints that provided movement for artificial limbs. This new development aided knights, who needed workable arms and legs for battle. Samples of artificial limbs from this period can be seen in the Stibbert Museum in Florence, Italy. One artificial

(Opposite page) An engraving depicts a worker at a lathe shaping a wooden bolt into an artificial leg. Early artificial limbs served as little more than crude replacements for lost or damaged arms and legs.

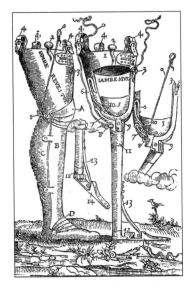

French surgeon Ambroise Paré designed this artificial leg in 1561. A metal casing covers a jointed knee and movable foot.

leg made for a knight has an armorlike outer covering with jointed knees and a movable foot—all operated by a string attached to a belt. Artificial arms, also of metal, have jointed wrists and elbows. In some cases the fingers are in a fixed, unbendable position. Other designs include movable fingers controlled by inner gears or a hinged mechanism.

Early artificial limbs such as these were heavy, bulky, and difficult to operate. Wooden legs had steel knee joints and wooden ankle joints that worked with cords attached to a belt worn around the waist. These human-made limbs were terribly uncomfortable.

Problems with limb attachments

Pain and soreness caused by the attachment of the limbs were a problem yet to be solved. People believed that the longer the body stump, the more adaptable it would be to an artificial limb. Surgeons tried to preserve as much of the natural arm or leg as possible when amputating. However, this created problems for the makers of artificial limbs. Limb makers believed that an ideal stump was one that was long enough to provide ample leverage for the artificial limb, yet short enough to avoid difficulties that develop when the end of the stump extends too close to the next joint.

Wearers of artificial limbs reported circulatory troubles and discomfort in thousands of case histories. Ill-fitting artificial limbs sometimes necessitated a second amputation. All of these problems showed a need for closer cooperation between the surgeon and the limb maker, preferably before amputation. The slow-developing artificial-limb technology served through several centuries and wars. However, those who lost limbs in the twentieth century would benefit from the knowledge gained from the past. The process of constructing and fitting artificial limbs became more refined. The next step would be to improve the materials used in making these appliances.

Materials and devices

In the early 1900s wood proved to be the best material for making artificial legs. Experiments using rawhide and leather failed because these materials soon lost their shape. Later, aluminum was used because of its strength and lightness. But it would be a long time before most amputees would be comfortable with their artificial limbs.

One man who had lost both arms astonished surgeons at the International Surgical Congress in New York with a demonstration of his artificial limbs. The demonstration was described in the July 31, 1915, *Literary Digest*. The man's arms were made of wood, with steel joints and rawhide

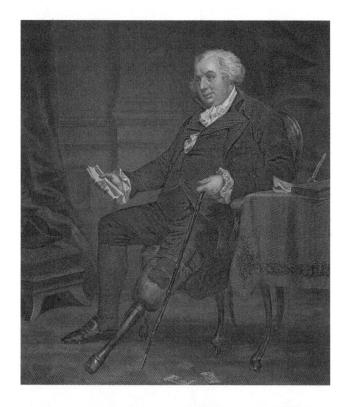

Some prostheses do not look like natural limbs. The peg leg was not attractive, but it was functional.

A worker measures and shapes
an artificial leg in an early
twentieth-century German
factory.

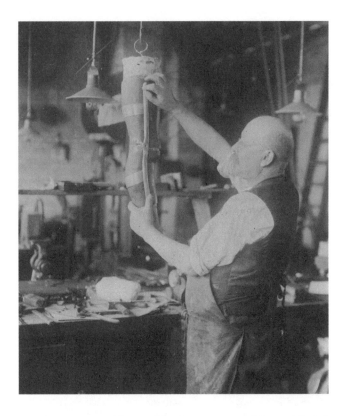

cord muscles. He wore gloves over his artificial
hands and showed how he was able to dress himself. He buttoned his shirt, tied a scarf and fastened it with a pin, then put on his coat and hat.
Next, he lit a cigarette, drew himself a drink from
a watercooler without spilling a drop, and wrote
his name. The article went on to describe the amputee's artificial arms, how they were attached to
his body, and how the wearer made them move:

> The arms are made of willow-fiber, with rawhide
> cords as muscles, each one attached to suspenders
> stretched across the back and chest, to give ten-
> sion. Forward movement of the stump raises the
> elbow. A downward movement of the shoulder
> pulls the finger-cord, bending the hand backward
> from the wrist joint and opening the fingers. An-
> other shrug of the shoulder closes the fingers and
> locks them so that they can hold whatever object is
> being handled.

Although this man demonstrated remarkable dexterity, most early artificial limb wearers were not as successful. The belts, straps, and tight-fitting undergarments, called corsets, used to secure limbs remained bulky and heavy and bothersome. Most wearers gave up and abandoned their artificial limbs. The limb makers continued to strive for better, more usable replacement organs.

Great improvements were reported in a 1918 issue of *The World's Work*. New devices such as hooks, rotating wrist sockets, and fake hands with movable thumbs and fingers made good substitutes for real hands. These parts were detachable at the wrist. Whatever tool fit the job in question would fit into the wrist socket. These devices made it possible for amputees to work in many occupations. Field laborers could use a ringed hook to grip a spade or hoe. Mechanics used a pivoting socket to clamp and hold tools. Steel hooks could be arranged to work in opposition, similar to the thumb and fingers of a real hand. For professions that required writing or drawing tools, a hand with fingers in a partially flexed position and a movable thumb controlled by muscles of the upper arm and shoulder was available. Some artificial hands even had jointed fingers with fake fingernails.

Despite improvements it was still tedious for an arm amputee to master the biceps, or shoulder action, necessary to flex and extend mechanically operated wrists, fingers, and thumbs. However, with determination and patience, it was feasible for an armless person to learn to do things that previously seemed impossible.

Wars stimulate joint improvement

The wars in the twentieth century gave added urgency to the manufacturing and improvement of artificial limbs. Hundreds of thousands of soldiers were maimed in battle. They lost their limbs—either through amputation or from explosions caused by land mines, grenades, and other weapons.

In a combined effort military hospitals all over the world worked tirelessly toward helping these maimed soldiers resume a normal life. Civilians wearing artificial limbs were brought to military hospitals to demonstrate walking, running, dancing, and boxing. It was hoped that witnessing these achievements would instill confidence in the amputees and show them that determination and practice could lead to success.

Determination was what Charles C. McGonegal had. McGonegal's success story spanning twenty-six years was reported in the November 25, 1944, *Saturday Evening Post.* In 1918, during World War I, McGonegal lost both hands when a grenade he was holding exploded. After three years of wearing cosmetic, limited-functioning hands, which had spring fingers with rubber tips

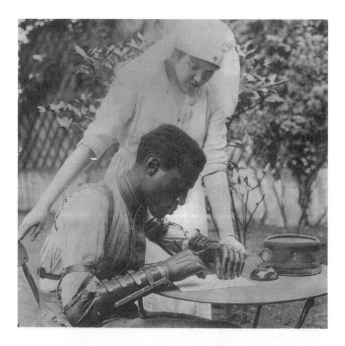

A Red Cross nurse stands by while a Senegalese man with two artificial arms writes a letter in 1918.

covered by a glove, McGonegal abandoned them for steel utility hooks. Though the hooks were discomforting for other people to look at, McGonegal found them to be more useful. Through many hours of practice with his hooks, McGonegal learned to use knives, forks, spoons, and coffee cups, as well as to fasten buttons, draw, and write. He and another soldier, Walter Antoniewicz, a leg amputee, teamed up to visit army and navy amputation centers across the United States.

Bringing hope to thousands

During these hospital visits McGonegal and Antoniewicz brought hope to thousands of young men who had lost legs and arms in the war. Their informal talks were laced with humor. Antoniewicz displayed the pinup pictures painted on his willow-wood legs and the thumbtack he used to hold his socks up. These demonstrations always got a laugh and made the amputees see that the time might come when they, too, could have a sense of humor about their predicament. Other countries wanted their veterans to use artificial limbs successfully, also. Canada met its obligation to its seven hundred amputation cases with thoroughness and speed. The May 18, 1918, *Scientific American* reported Canada's attitude:

> A new light has been shed on the subject [amputees and disabled], with the result that nations no longer look upon the loss of an arm or leg or both eyes as the termination of a man's productive career. Instead of pensioning off the crippled soldier as was formerly the practice, the new order of things calls for the reconstruction of that human wreck, in order that sooner or later he may be returned to normal life, ready and fit to fill some useful function in the workaday world.

The Canadian Military Hospitals Commission accepted responsibility to provide the required artificial limbs and keep them in good repair during the lifetime of the soldier. The commission provided the best artificial arms and legs yet invented anywhere in the world.

Construction and fitting

Canadian artificial legs were made of willow taken from the brittle willow and the golden osier trees, both originally grown in Europe, but now plentiful in the United States and Canada. Willow wood was used because it was tough, easy to work with, and did not split readily. It was cut into pieces, or bolts, twenty-two inches long and bored through the center in order for the wood to harden. The bark was removed, the ends painted, and the bolts were then left to season in the open

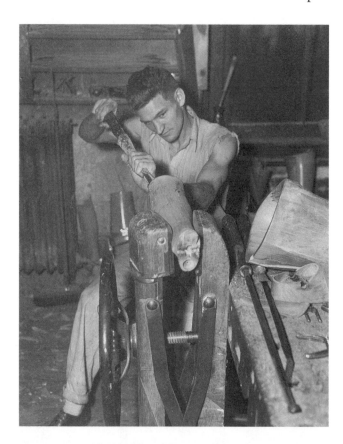

A Washington, D.C., plant made limbs for soldiers injured in the Spanish Civil War. In this 1938 photo a worker hollows out a wooden bolt.

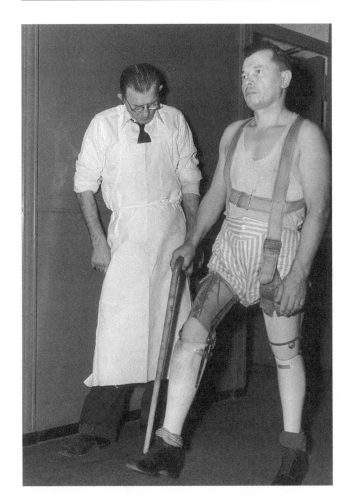

A doctor checks the final fit of an amputee's artificial legs. Belts and straps were used by 1939 to attach artificial limbs to remaining stumps.

air for two years. After seasoning, the bolts were kiln dried and stocked in various sizes.

Fitting an amputee with an artificial limb required several stages. First, the patient was measured. Then a limb was chosen. The top of the artificial leg was hollowed out to fit the stump. But this was only a rough facsimile of what the artificial leg would be by the time the patient left the hospital. While still at the hospital, the patient walked with the crude leg. The leg continued to be trimmed until it fit comfortably. The next stage was to hollow out the leg as thinly as possible. Wet rawhide was then glued to the outside to keep the wood from splitting. The exterior was covered with paint, while the interior surface got a coat of shiny wood-oil varnish. The final step was fitting a boot to the artificial foot. No limb was considered complete until maximum comfort and every desirable feature available had been obtained for the amputee. If the artificial limb did not fit the stump comfortably, it would be adjusted as many times as necessary.

By 1916 artificial arms and legs looked and performed like the real thing. Those who were legless and armless could now climb ladders, use delicate tools, and play musical instruments. Some amputees were concerned about the appearance of their hooks and were embarrassed to wear them for social occasions. In that case the hook could be exchanged for a gloved hand with a workable thumb.

Furnishing artificial limbs for war victims and other disabled people and rehabilitating these people to restore their earning power was a priority for all nations. In the United States a law was passed in 1920 that required all states to provide rehabilitation programs for war victims. Eventually these rehabilitation programs were incorporated into the federal Social Security Act. By 1937 constructing artificial limbs was a six-million-dollar industry in the United States.

Limb wearers

Within that industry, 58 percent of the manufacturers wore artificial limbs themselves. *Time* magazine's October 18, 1937, issue reported activities at the Association of Limb Manufacturers convention. The amputees not only discussed serious problems, but they had fun demonstrating the capabilities of their artificial limbs in such difficult tasks as dancing, skipping rope, and knotting neckties. Showing a sense of humor, one

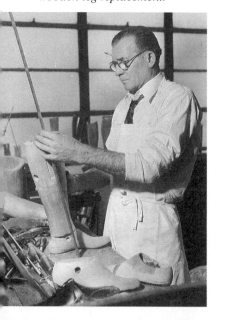

A 1939 photograph shows a limb maker measuring a carved wooden leg replacement.

manufacturer, Joe Spievak, who had lost both legs at age seventeen, told about two advantages of artificial legs: "Your feet do not perspire and you do not have to change socks often." Another man, Clyde Aunger, who lost a leg in a trolley car accident at age sixteen, proudly revealed a music box in the calf of his artificial wooden leg.

By that time materials used in artificial limbs had greatly improved. About 80 percent of artificial limbs were made from willow or aluminum. An adult artificial arm weighed about five pounds and could be attached in two or three minutes. A natural arm of a 180-pound man weighs approximately seven pounds in comparison. At that time most artificial limbs functioned for about five or six years before they needed to be replaced.

Even though early replacements for body parts were crude, they progressed to looking more life-like and to being more functional. Crude as these artificial organs were, they made life more enjoyable for many people. Encouraged, scientists began working on aids for defective internal organs.

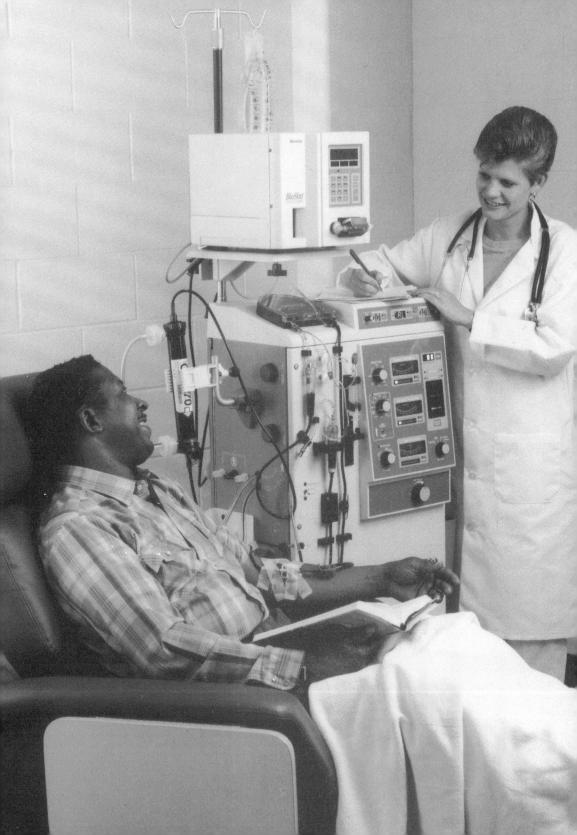

2

The Kidney: First Internal Organ to Use Machine Assistance

(Opposite page) Although the artificial kidney does the work of an internal organ, it performs that job from outside the body. During hemodialysis treatment the artificial kidney cleanses waste from a patient's blood, a process that takes about four hours.

THE ARTIFICIAL KIDNEY, also known as a dialyzer, was first used successfully on a patient in 1943. It represented a huge breakthrough in artificial-organ technology because it marked the first time a defective internal organ was assisted by human-made parts. Although the dialyzer was still an external machine, visible to the eye, like an artificial arm or leg, it aided an organ inside the body cavity.

The artificial kidney accomplishes two specific functions that the diseased kidneys can no longer do. It balances the fluid and chemicals in the body and excretes, or eliminates, waste products. In the past when the kidneys failed, the patient died from the poisonous waste products that built up in the blood. People who lost kidney function had no chance for leading a normal life until dialysis became a reality.

Dialysis is a form of medical treatment that removes the body's wastes directly from the blood.

There are two forms of dialysis: hemodialysis, which uses an artificial kidney dialysis machine, and peritoneal dialysis, which uses the lining, or peritoneum, of the abdominal cavity. Dialysis does not cure kidney failure, but it does allow a person to maintain life and reasonable health.

Kidneys are the master chemists of the body. These fist-size organs in the lower back have many functions. They adjust the body's fluids, balance the body's chemicals, release several hormones, and remove waste products from the body. Removing waste products is done by purifying or filtering the blood, which is the kidneys' most important function. This buildup of waste is called urea and may act like poison in the body, creating a condition known as uremia. Long before an artificial kidney would be feasible, scientists experimented with an outside filter that could strain molecules from liquids. This filter mimicked the natural kidney's filtering system.

In 1913 at Johns Hopkins University, an experimental filtering system was tried on several dogs. Scientists John J. Abel, L. G. Rowntree, and B. B. Turner wanted to show that an acidic compound introduced into a dog's blood could be filtered out through thin tissue, or membrane, and the cleansed blood returned to the dog's body. The acidic compound chosen was aspirin, which simulated the poisons in the blood that are ordinarily filtered out through the kidney. The scientists used a transparent material called cellophane, invented in 1908, as the filtering membrane.

Cellophane was first used for the outer skin of sausages. It was thin and flexible and had microscopic pores that allowed passage of some substances. These characteristics made cellophane a good material for early efforts to copy the natural kidney filtering process.

In their experiments the scientists built a network of tubelike cellophane membranes. The membranes were submerged in a liquid bath. After giving a dog large doses of aspirin, they passed its blood through the submerged tubes, where the aspirin then filtered out into the liquid bath.

From the results of this and other similar experiments, the scientists theorized that poisoned human blood could also be filtered through a fine-pored membrane, which would strain out the waste product. The cleansed blood would be returned to the body. The results of these experiments with dogs formed the basis for later artificial-kidney research and the invention of the artificial kidney.

The work of Willem J. Kolff

One of the doctors who pursued the goal of building an artificial kidney was Willem J. Kolff. In medical wards in the Netherlands in 1938, Dr. Kolff saw the agony of kidney failure—high blood pressure, headaches, vomiting, and, ultimately, death. He became obsessed with the idea of reversing the disease. Author John G. Deaton, in *New Parts for Old*, quotes Kolff: "The idea grew in me that if we could only remove twenty grams of urea and other retention products per day, we might relieve this man's nausea and that, if we did this from day to day, life might still be possible." Kolff decided to test the theory demonstrated by the 1913 experiments of Abel, Rowntree, and Turner.

Kolff began his work by filling a section of cellophane sausage tubing with blood. He fastened the tube to a small board to give it stability. Next, Kolff immersed the board in a saltwater, or saline, bath. He added urea to the blood in the tube. For thirty minutes Kolff rocked the tube board back

Dr. Willem J. Kolff is credited with building the first successful model of the artificial kidney. It was first used on a patient in 1943.

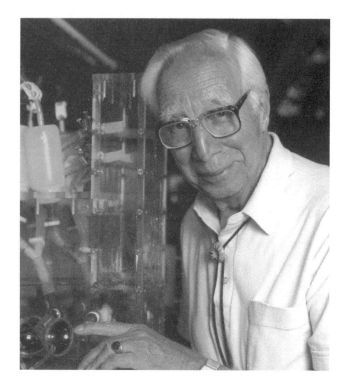

and forth in the saline bath to encourage the filtering process. Needed blood cells and protein could not pass through the cellophane into the surrounding saltwater because they were too large to get through the small pores in the cellophane. But the urea, salt, potassium, and other waste products passed out of the blood, through the cellophane, and into the saline solution. This kind of separation through a membrane is called dialysis. The next step was to build a machine that could filter a human's blood in the same way.

Kolff did not discover the filtering process, or dialysis, nor was he the first to attempt to use this process to build an artificial kidney. Others had tried before Kolff, but he is given credit for building the first successful model. Author Janice M. Cauwels in *The Body Shop*, quotes Kolff:

> I am not really the inventor of the artificial kidney. The artificial kidney was described by Abel,

Rowntree and Turner, three Americans, in the City of Groningen, The Netherlands, during a Physiological Congress in 1913. I was two years old at that time, and I do not remember it, but in that same city I began to work on artificial kidneys in 1939.

Building the artificial kidney

Kolff had built several artificial kidneys by 1940. None of these dialyzers worked well enough to use on patients. But he was on the right track. His work was interrupted in May 1940 when the Germans invaded the Netherlands during World War II.

To aid people wounded in the bombing, Kolff set up a blood bank. Operating the blood bank proved useful in his progress toward building a successful artificial kidney. Working with tubes of blood outside of the body, he learned about the drug heparin, which kept blood from clotting. Heparin would prove helpful to use when blood passed through an artificial kidney.

Despite the war Kolff's experiments continued. By 1941 he had moved to the tiny Dutch town of Kampen. At the municipal hospital Kolff worked in secrecy during the Nazi occupation. He often hid his equipment so the Nazis would not take it away from him.

Kolff built his first rotating model of an artificial kidney in secret, using parts built by a local manufacturer. This device had no pump. Instead, the patient's blood was drawn into a glass container that was repeatedly raised to the ceiling on a pulley. From there the blood drained into a rotating drum, where it circulated through the tubing. He made eight artificial kidneys, often scrounging for materials and buying them himself.

By March 1943 Kolff had improved his dialysis machine with an electric motor and was ready

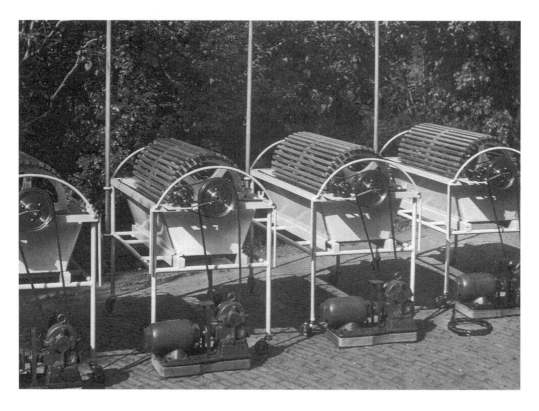

These first rotating dialyzers, or artificial kidneys, were built by Dr. Kolff in the Netherlands in 1944. When World War II ended they were shipped to other countries.

to try it on a human. Kolff's dialysis machine measured about two feet wide, four feet long, and three feet high. The machine consisted of twenty yards of cellophane tubing wrapped around an aluminum drum. Immersed in a salt-solution bath, inside an enamel tank, this drum was turned by an electric motor. The patient's blood entered the cellophane tubing. The drum, half-filled with a clear rinsing solution, or dialysis fluid, revolved slowly. Gravity propelled the blood and dialysis fluid to the lowest part of the drum while urea and other wastes flowed out through the cellophane tubing. Then the cleansed blood was returned to the body.

One problem Kolff had to correct was the leaking at the connections where the blood entered and left the cylinder. Kolff knew that the Ford Motor Company made good-quality seals for the water pumps in its engines. He visited the local Ford dealer to see how the seals were made and then duplicated their procedure on his cylinder.

Human experiments

With this problem solved, Kolff was anxious to test the artificial kidney on patients suffering with fatal kidney disease. He began his tests on March 17, 1943. The first patient was a twenty-nine-year-old woman suffering from kidney failure and other medical problems that accompany kidney disease. Author Thomas Metos, in *Artificial Humans*, describes the treatment:

> She received twelve dialysis treatments. At first, the blood was drawn from the patient in a small amount, placed in the artificial kidney for dialysis, and then reinjected into the patient to see if any serious reactions would take place. When no serious reactions occurred, larger and larger amounts of blood were dialyzed, until almost six quarts of blood were being dialyzed. During the last treatments, the blood was continuously fed into, and returned from, the artificial kidney by tube. Later, a pump was used to circulate the blood from patient to machine and back again. Then a permanent connection made of glass was inserted into one of the patient's arteries for the transfer of blood.

Despite the treatment, that first patient died. Over the next thirty months fifteen more near-death patients were treated with artificial kidneys. All died. However, Kolff's seventeenth patient, who started treatment on September 11, 1945, recovered completely. She was a sixty-seven-year-old woman who lived many years after her recovery from acute renal, or kidney, failure. Others treated with the artificial kidney came out of their comas. One patient recovered consciousness long enough to write his will. Thus, Kolff knew the blood dialysis had helped. Author Cauwels quotes Kolff during this human trial of the artificial kidney: "I was tired and desperate at times. We had to work during the day and dialyze at night. It took at least six hours, so often I didn't get home until dawn. On one occasion I was so overtired that I cried and cried."

In order to continue his work on the dialysis machines, Kolff persisted in experimenting with dialysis fluids and drugs like heparin. By 1945 he had built eight more machines. After the war news of Kolff's invention spread, and he began giving his artificial kidney machines to scientists and physicians in other countries. His machine became the model for all others built after it. In May 1947 Kolff was invited to New York City, where he detailed his work on the artificial kidney to American doctors in a meeting at Mount Sinai Hospital.

In 1950 Kolff accepted a position at the Cleveland Clinic Foundation in Ohio. At the clinic Kolff established the world's first department of artificial organs and opened the doors for the development of other artificial organs. Kolff also continued his work on the artificial kidney, finding ways to make it smaller, portable, and disposable.

An aid for frequent dialysis users

Until 1960 most doctors believed the artificial kidney could be used as a substitute when the natural kidney experienced temporary failure. They did not consider the artificial kidney a practical solution to long-term failure because blood-vessel surgery was required each time the patient was hooked up to an artificial kidney. Surgery involved inserting tubes, one each in an artery and a vein. The tubes carried the blood to and from the equipment. No more than a dozen such operations were feasible. Therefore, successful treatment was confined to patients whose own kidneys could resume working in a few weeks.

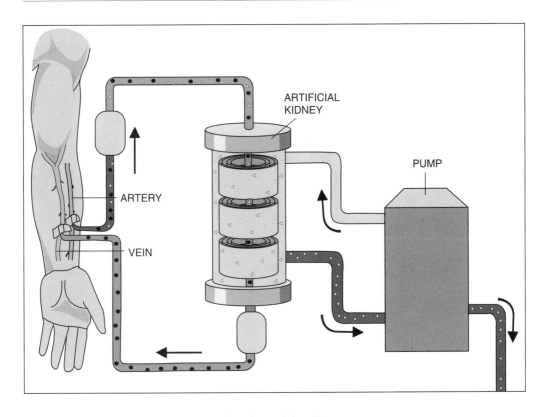

The hemodialysis process shows impure blood flowing out of the artery into a compartment surrounded by dialysis fluid. Here it is cleansed and returned to the body via the vein.

Then a new technique was developed by Dr. Belding H. Scribner at the University of Washington School of Medicine in Seattle. It allowed an unlimited number of blood-cleansing treatments. The new technique was to permanently implant a set of tubes into the forearm. One tube was threaded into an artery, the other into a vein. The tubes could be left in place for about a year or longer, as long as the tubes did not plug up or become infected. The implanted tubes were connected by an exterior U-shaped tube, called a shunt, to maintain normal circulation. When it was time for a treatment, the shunt was removed, and the artificial kidney was connected to the two implanted tubes. The patient was simply plugged in, making it possible to have multiple treatments without undergoing blood-vessel surgery each time.

Patients who have permanent kidney malfunction must receive dialysis for the rest of their lives or until they receive a kidney transplant. The dialysis procedure is painless, and patients can read, watch television, or sleep during treatments.

Not enough artificial kidneys

By 1966 there were fifty-seven dialysis centers across the country. However, these centers could accommodate only five hundred Americans with incurable kidney disease. More centers were needed. A 1970 statistic stated that sixty thousand Americans died of some kind of kidney disease annually. About half died because of lack of money for treatment or lack of the availability of kidney machines. Due to the high cost of the kidney machines and the scarcity of trained staff to operate them, many people were turned away from treatment and died. The annual cost of treating a single patient was about twenty-five thousand dollars.

The limited number of dialysis facilities forced doctors and others to choose who would live and who would die. At most centers a group of local citizens and physicians screened candidates and used family size and patient age to help make the decision. In the July 25, 1966, *Newsweek* one panel member was quoted: "We are aware we are voting against a person's opportunity to live. This would be unbearable if you knew the person and had to see him face to face."

In an article in the November 1967 *Redbook*, a medical director described the predicament:

> Right now we can't dialyze everyone who might be helped by dialysis because we simply haven't got the trained personnel to do the job and the money to buy machines we need. As a result people have to die. I know it's tragic to realize that this is happening in the twentieth century when we're trying to send a man to the moon. But I feel I'm helpless. I wish there were some easy solution.

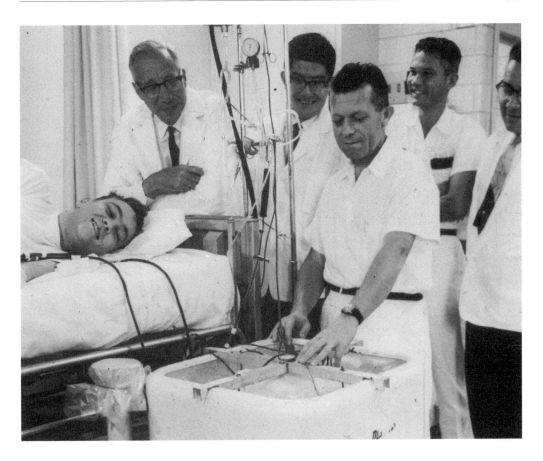

The solution was to develop smaller machines that could fit in the home and to train family members to operate the equipment. Kolff and Cleveland Clinic Foundation associates developed a simple home-use artificial kidney. Dr. Kolff described the fifteen-hundred-dollar annual home treatment in the February 4, 1967, issue of *Business Week*:

Dr. Willem Kolff (standing, left) and associates observe washing-machine dialysis at the Cleveland Clinic.

> It uses a Maytag washing machine, without the wringer; . . . it uses inexpensive cellophane for the filtering unit at a cost of about sixteen cents per dialysis "run" and it employs pre-packaged chemicals which, when mixed with warm tap water, serve as the machine's cleansing solution.

The treatment required two months of training for patients at the Cleveland Clinic. There are drawbacks to this method if the patient cannot learn to perform at-home dialysis or keep the equipment sterile. "However," Kolff said, "it boils down to a choice between bankruptcy, death, and do-it-yourself."

By 1972, 40 percent of the four thousand Americans on kidney machines treated themselves at home. Yet even with home treatments available, many patients were too frightened to use them. And many family members were afraid they would be responsible for a loved one's death.

Government help

Because of these fears many people continued to die from kidney disease. In order to halt the great number of deaths from renal failure, the National Kidney Foundation lobbied for years for funds to aid dying kidney patients. Finally, in 1973 Congress passed a bill that allowed long-term, or chronic, renal disease patients to receive benefits for dialysis and transplants. With monetary support from the government, kidney patients did not have to die. Three years later the March 7, 1976, *New York Times Magazine* quoted a hospital administrator about the success of the congressional bill: "We were keeping people at work. We were keeping families together."

By the 1980s scientists developed a new artificial kidney for young people that replaced in-hospital machines. The process uses the body's own peritoneal membrane, or abdominal cavity lining, to do the dialyzing. A tube called a catheter is surgically implanted in the abdomen. Sterile fluids drain into the cavity and drain out four hours later, carrying waste products from the blood with them. The daytime continuous ambulatory peritoneal dialysis (CAPD) and nighttime continuous cycling peritoneal dialysis (CCPD)

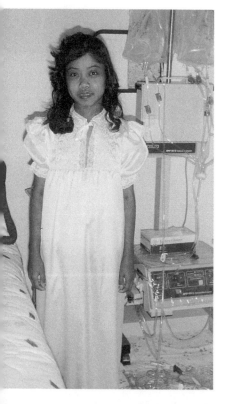

Joyce Roscel Joaquin is shown in her bedroom next to her home dialysis machine. For ten hours each night, while she sleeps, reads, or watches TV, Joyce's blood is cleansed by continuous cycling peritoneal dialysis (CCPD).

treatments offer an alternative to thrice-weekly, four-to-five-hour hemodialysis treatments at a dialysis center. No longer confined to hospitals or treatment centers, children and young adults can attend school and engage in other activities by using the peritoneal dialysis system.

Dialysis centers worldwide

Over three hundred different types of artificial kidneys are now available worldwide. An estimated half a million patients are on dialysis, of which 20 percent use the peritoneal dialysis method. Hemodialysis centers exist worldwide, enabling patients who enjoy traveling to do so.

By the 1950s scientists were working on how to replace many internal organs, not just the kidney. However, a big part of the challenge of developing internal artificial organs was finding materials that the body would not reject.

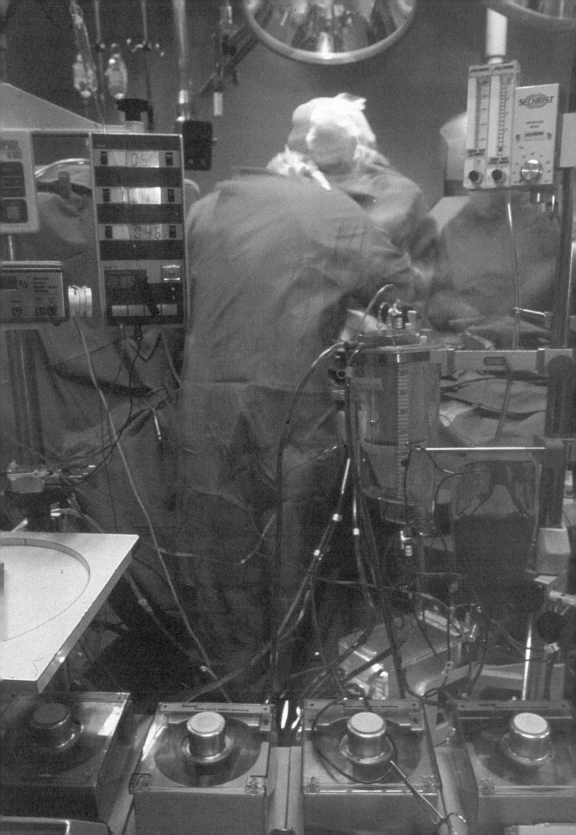

3

Vessels, Valves, and Heart-Assist Devices

IMPLANTABLE MATERIALS THAT the human body would tolerate were difficult to develop. The human body is like a chemical swamp—with acids, salts, and antibodies, which seek out and attack foreign materials. It is an unfriendly environment for implants. Some materials, like wood, are not tolerated inside the body. However, many types of metal, plastic, and glass are acceptable.

The human body can do one of three things with implanted foreign material: accept it, break it apart, or reject it. Therefore, materials used for inner artificial organs must combine antirejection, wear resistance, and environmental survival qualities. These materials are known as biomaterials. Some of the most useful biomaterials are metals, ceramics, and polymers, or plastics. Materials that come in contact with flowing blood have additional requirements. They must not damage the blood cells nor encourage the blood to clot. Nonliving materials have to bond to living surfaces inside the body to create successful implants.

Once these biomaterials were developed and available, procedures to replace deteriorating

(Opposite page) The heart-lung machine in the foreground does the work of the heart and lungs during surgery. It allows doctors to perform cardiac surgery in a bloodless area.

inner-body parts with human-made parts progressed rapidly. These included a heart-lung machine for use in surgeries, artificial or synthetic valves, development of a pacemaker to keep the heart beating rhythmically, and synthetic arteries. Creating synthetic arteries presented an especially difficult challenge.

Blood flow must not be obstructed

From the beginning of the twentieth century, surgical researchers had tried to find durable substitutes to replace worn-out arteries. They used many different materials while trying to construct workable tubes: metal, glass, plastic, pieces of patients' own veins, arteries from deceased donors, even strips of nylon petticoat stitched into tube shapes.

Because blood flowing through the body keeps a person alive, it is important that the blood circulates smoothly and uninterrupted. Vessels, veins, and arteries are all tubes that perform this function. Unfortunately, sometimes they wear out or plug up and need to be replaced.

Artery replacement began in 1903 when German scientist E. Hopfer made the first successful transplant of arteries from one dog to another. Dr. Alexis Carrel, of the Rockefeller Institute for Medical Research, followed with a second dog-artery transplant in 1905. In 1948 Dr. Robert E. Gross, of Children's Hospital in Boston, used human artery transplants that were preserved in a special solution and refrigerated. But since the demand for arteries exceeded the supply, doctors continued to search for a strong artificial artery.

In the 1950s the busiest center that worked on faulty arteries was the Baylor University College of Medicine in Houston, which was headed by Dr. Michael E. DeBakey. Of DeBakey's forty aneurysm—burst or diseased vessel—surgeries,

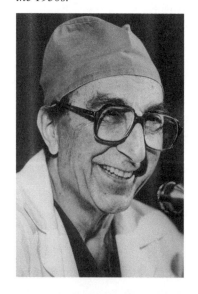

Dr. Michael E. DeBakey performed successful artificial vessel replacement surgeries in the 1950s.

two-thirds of the patients survived. At first donor vessels obtained from autopsies were used, but eventually synthetic arteries proved to be stronger and more immune to disease.

In creating artificial blood vessels, scientists faced the challenging problem of finding a fabric that would not be absorbed by body fluids. It needed to be strong, stretchy, and smooth, without loose fibers; it had to allow consistent blood flow and to be easily attached by using surgical suturing, or sewing, techniques.

At Columbia-Presbyterian Medical Center in New York, Drs. Arthur Blakemore, Arthur B. Voorhees Jr., and A. Jarotski III tried to form a seamed replacement tube by using fine-woven cloth. They first tested the fabric tube in a dog. The tube was sewn to the dog's main artery, called the aorta. Soon the dog's natural tissues lined the artificial artery with a smooth, solid layer of its own cells. This meant that the body had accepted the artificial vessel. Encouraged, surgeons began using the cloth artery in human patients in 1953.

The shoelace solution

At this point Chemstrand Corporation in Alabama, working on a nonprofit, public-service basis, became involved in developing synthetic arteries. Dr. James S. Tapp, head of Chemstrand's pioneering research section, patterned the first artifical arteries on the braided tubing design of nylon shoelaces. Experimenting with 250 yards of nylon shoelaces, he dipped the strands into a solution of formic acid to make the nylon firmer. Next, Dr. Tapp treated the nylon with silicone to make it water-resistant.

For his experiments Tapp purchased the braided nylon tubing in larger diameters—one-quarter to three-quarters of an inch. The tubing was tested in dogs' aortas as well as in the groin

*Crinkled artificial arteries
replace clogged or burst vessels
to provide for a free flow of
blood throughout the body.*

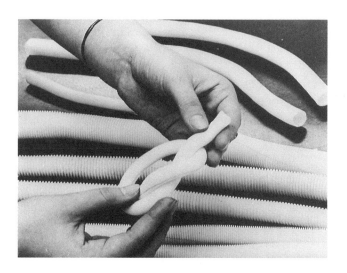

of a human patient. But these first nylon arteries did not work well because they kinked when bent, and that shut off the blood flow.

This problem was solved by accident. Tapp happened to push a length of braided nylon tubing off a glass rod, and the tubing crinkled into accordion pleats, like a paper wrapper does when removed from a drinking straw. When he tried bending the wrinkled tubing, its central passage stayed open. It was kink-proof!

Heat treatments set the pleats permanently. The crimped tube worked well on a dog's aorta, with the dog's tissue lining the tube to give blood a smooth, nonclotting flow. The pleats also gave the synthetic artery flexibility for stretching over hip and knee joints. Another artificial artery was developed in Houston by Dr. DeBakey. It was a knitted Dacron artery. The Dacron arteries were made on a modified forty-year-old necktie knitting machine.

Before insertion, the fabric arteries contained thousands of tiny holes. Once inside the body, the holes became sealed by the patient's coagulating blood. Cell tissue formed around and grew through the fabric tubing. It was as though the substitute part had always belonged where it was placed. In effect, the body took over and actually possessed the human-made blood vessel as its own. The artificial blood vessels saved the lives of many people.

Problems with natural blood vessels

Natural blood-carrying vessels can become infected, injured, hardened, or stretched very thin. When an artery is stretched thin, it generally balloons out like a weak spot in a bicycle tire tube. It can burst, and the victim may bleed to death. This is known as an aneurysm and can happen in the aorta, which is the main trunk of arteries that carries blood to all organs except the lungs.

Thinning blood vessels are not the only problem. Vessels may also get clogged and become very narrow, decreasing blood flow. This narrowing of the blood vessels provokes pain in the legs, cramping, and extreme fatigue when walking. Sometimes a nylon implant is inserted to bypass the obstructed segments of blood vessels. Most blood circulatory problems can be solved with artificial blood vessels. Today there is scarcely a spot along the main channels of the body's bloodstream that surgeons cannot reach for repairs.

A machine that works like the heart

However, the easy access to the arteries was not duplicated when it came to reaching flawed parts of the heart. Because of the amount of blood present, it was difficult for surgeons to even see what they were doing, much less worry about interrupting the blood flow through the heart.

At the University of Minnesota a group of scientists headed by Dr. Clarence Dennis developed the heart-lung machine in 1949. The heart-lung machine was a device that did the complex job of both the heart, which pumps the blood, and the

This 1950 heart-lung machine is composed of a pump and an oxygenator which temporarily acts as the patient's heart and lungs during surgery.

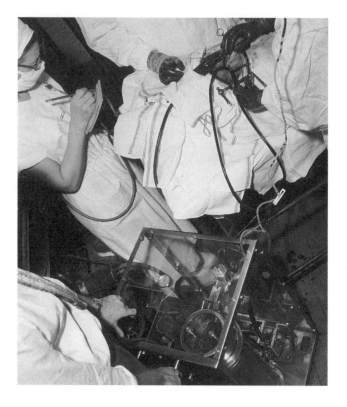

lungs, which add oxygen to the blood, without damaging the blood itself. The machine could be used during heart surgery to give the surgeon a dry work area for as long as thirty to sixty minutes, enabling work to proceed without blood obscuring the view. This so-called iron heart had two principal parts: a pump for circulating blood, and an oxygenator. The oxygenator supplied oxygen to the circulating blood and also removed carbon dioxide.

A leaky heart valve is like a leaky faucet

Once the surgeons could perform surgery on the heart parts, another important part of the heart—the valves—could be repaired or replaced. A valve is a membranous structure that prevents the return flow of a fluid. Doctors compare damaged valves to leaky faucets. There are four valves in the heart that allow the flow of blood into a heart chamber. If the valve, which consists of two or three flaps of limp tissue, does not shut completely or impedes the passage of blood, it can cause cardiac (heart) or circulatory illness.

The aortic valve is one of four valves that guide the flow of blood through the four chambers of the heart. An artificial valve must assure a free forward flow of blood and prevent leakage back into the heart. Most aortic valve problems are caused by rheumatic fever, a childhood disease that leaves scar tissue on the heart valves. Replacing the defective valves depended on finding the right materials to make a valve that would perform as well as the natural valve.

The Starr-Edwards valve

In 1957 a retired aerospace engineer, M. Lowell Edwards, began working with heart surgeon Dr. Albert Starr of the University of Oregon Medical School. Together they worked to develop a better artificial heart valve than the unsatisfactory valve being used at that time. The engineer had to build a valve that would withstand one hundred thousand daily openings and closings. The valve also had to be accurate in regulating the flow of fluid through the sixty thousand miles of arteries, veins, and capillaries in the human body. As an engineer, Edwards believed he could contribute to medicine. Already an inventor of equipment related to aircraft, pulp, and paper, Edwards went to work on the valve.

The Starr-Edwards valve was not created in a modern laboratory, but in Edwards's backyard toolshed. Starr and Edwards spent two and a half years testing various materials and experimenting with animals. At last, in 1960 the Starr-Edwards valve was ready for a final test. Instead of the natural flap-type valve, their valve was a silicone ball enclosed in a cage. In order to test the new valve, the scientists used an accelerated test pump. The pump working the valve would be sped up in order to simulate the equivalent of forty-three years of wear in the human heart. The model valve was subjected to 750 times the normal stress—opening and closing at a rate of six thousand times a minute. Over a three-week period the ball retained its shape, dimension, and weight. The Starr-Edwards valve was first implanted in a human in September 1960.

The patient was a fifty-two-year-old man whose heart had been scarred and deformed by rheumatic fever. Since the patient lived several years after surgery, the new valve was considered a success.

After almost four years and twenty-six hundred implants of the Starr-Edwards valve, Dr. Starr reported in the January 1964 issue of *Today's Health*:

> The artificial heart valve is here to stay. Our job is not to design a valve identical to nature's, not to see how close we can come to duplicating a natural phenomenon, but to overcome the clinical problem of the diseased heart valve. If we can do this with a valve similar to the natural one—fine. But we must evaluate on the basis of function, rather than form.

These Starr-Edwards valves were used to replace three heart valves—the aortic, mitral, and tricuspid. In the November 20, 1965, issue of *Science News Letter*, Dr. Starr estimated that ten thousand persons were wearing one or more valves. He noted that eight hundred to one thousand valves a month were being implanted in humans at a cost of $225 for each valve. "We do not claim that the valves are perfect," Dr. Starr said. "Sometimes a temporary speech block occurs even if the operation is successful, but we are continually trying to perfect the parts."

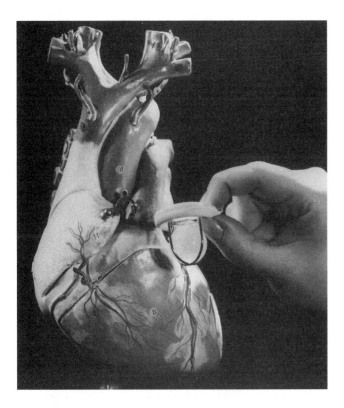

Not all surgeons favored metal or plastic devices for valve replacements. In 1966 two surgeons, Sir Russell Brock, director of cardiology at Guy's Hospital in London, England, and Dr. Charles P. Bailey of Saint Barnabas Hospital in New York, insisted that human or animal tissue should be used instead of artificial materials. They believed that either a patient's own tissue or that from a deceased person was superior, since the shape of the flaps was more natural than the ball in a cage. They cautioned enthusiastic surgeons not to be blinded to the possibility of using tissue instead of synthetic parts. Some physicians favored using pig valves to replace human valves. Pig valves are superior to valves made of synthetic materials because they cause less clotting.

All of these theories are probably correct. However, more patients could be served with synthetic valves because of availability. With artificial heart valves being used to control the flow of blood, another problem could also be solved artificially. This is the heart's ability to regulate the pumping of blood in a rhythmic fashion.

Electricity gives the heart rhythm

The heart's natural pacemaker keeps the rhythm of the heartbeat by passing electrical signals from the auricle to the ventricle chambers, which allows blood to be pumped through the body. When this pace is interrupted, it is called heart block.

Doctors searched for a device that could be used to restore the heartbeat. In 1952 Drs. Paul M. Zoll and Leona R. Norman of Boston's Beth Israel Hospital perfected a machine that could either restore the heartbeat or speed it up. The machine accomplished this by giving the heart muscle electric shocks at frequencies between

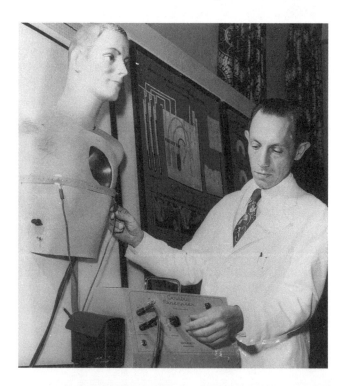

Dr. Paul Zoll uses a dummy to demonstrate the cardiac pacemaker machine which restores a rhythmic heartbeat to a defective heart.

fifty and one hundred a minute. Normally the heart rate is seventy to eighty beats a minute.

The machine was called a cardiac pacemaker and had to be operated in the hospital. The fifteen-pound machine used two flat metal electrodes that were attached to the patient's exterior chest wall. Because the machine administered distinct shocks, it could not be applied longer than an hour. It also burned the skin.

Improving the pacemaker

By 1957 a heart surgeon at the University of Minnesota, Dr. C. Walton Lellehei, along with two engineers, developed a pocket-size transistorized pacemaker. This model, which gave the wearer hospital-free independence, was worn attached to the waist area. Two bare ends of braided stainless-steel wires, insulated with a silicone plastic, were embedded into a ventricle. The wires exited through a small hole in the chest wall and were attached to the pacemaker, which was about the size of a deck of cards. The device electronically stimulated the heart to beat at a normal rate. Although this equipment was life saving, the protruding wires and terminal box were cumbersome and made everyday tasks an effort, especially bathing.

By 1960 a new silicone-rubber-coated internal pacemaker was designed and built by Drs. William Chardack and Andrew Gage, and engineer Wilson Greatbatch. The two-and-one-half-inch device was small enough to be sewn under the skin at just about the belt line, with inner wires leading to the heart. Although the patient needed surgery every three to five years to replace batteries, the resulting freedom was liberating to users. Surgeons and engineers would next strive toward replacing other worn-out heart parts and, ultimately, the heart itself.

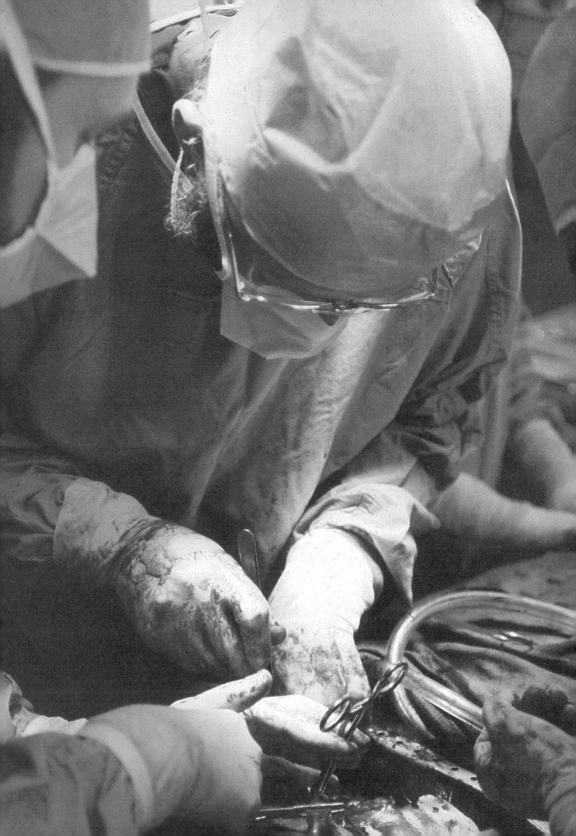

4

The Artificial Heart

SCIENTISTS DEVOTED THEMSELVES first to studying the function of bodily organs and then to duplicating these functions by artificial means. Their next goal, following the artificial vessels, heart-lung machine, valves, and heart pacemaker, was to develop an artificial heart. This device would be placed inside the body as a substitute for a natural heart that was too damaged for surgical repair.

However, a new set of technical problems arose. The problems were mechanical, electrical, and chemical. These three types of problems were more often solved by industrial scientists, who specialized in machines and motors, than by doctors. So medical scientists, who were familiar with the workings of the human body, blended their knowledge with that of the industrial scientists. This marriage of medical and industrial science brought about new developments in heart-related devices, such as pumps and compressors, and would eventually lead to the ultimate in artificial organs—a total replacement for the human heart.

The heart is the one organ in the body that is always working. It is fist-size, weighs about ten

(Opposite page) Permanent artificial hearts and heart boosters were tested in dogs and calves for about fifteen years before being implanted into humans. Here surgeons implant an artificial heart into an animal.

51

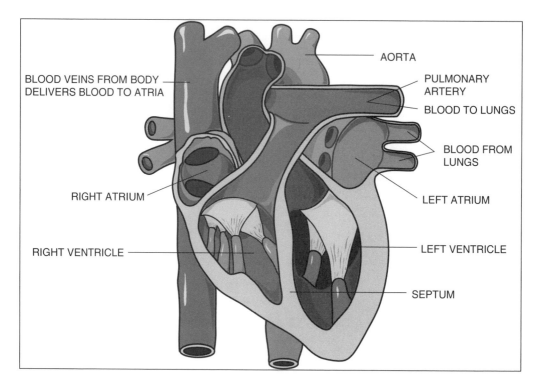

BLOOD VEINS FROM BODY DELIVERS BLOOD TO ATRIA

AORTA

PULMONARY ARTERY

BLOOD TO LUNGS

BLOOD FROM LUNGS

RIGHT ATRIUM

LEFT ATRIUM

RIGHT VENTRICLE

LEFT VENTRICLE

SEPTUM

ounces, is made mostly of muscle, and is located in the center of the chest. The heart muscle is divided into four hollow chambers that contain blood.

The heart is a pump that contracts and forces blood through vessels throughout the body—blood that contains oxygen, nutrients, and waste products. The blood is circulated around the body once each minute.

Each side of the heart has two chambers: an atrium, also known as an auricle, and a ventricle. The atrium, or upper chamber, receives blood through the veins. When the atrium contracts, it empties the blood through a one-way valve into the ventricle, or lower chamber. From the ventricle the blood is pumped out of the heart through the arteries to other parts of the body.

Divided by a wall called the septum, the right and left sides of the heart have two different jobs.

The right side takes in used, deoxygenated blood and pumps it through the pulmonary artery to the lungs. From the lungs the fresh, oxygen-rich blood flows into the left side of the heart. From the left ventricle, which is the largest and strongest chamber, the blood is pumped out through the aorta to the whole body.

When the heart beats, both atria contract at the same time, squeezing blood into the ventricles. They relax and rest while both ventricles contract together, forcing blood out into the body. An efficient system of valves prevents the blood from flowing in the wrong direction.

Blending of medical and technical knowledge

The project to develop an artificial heart required cooperation between the industrial scientist and the medical scientist. One such partnership between industry and medicine was formed at the Cleveland Clinic in Ohio, where Dr. Willem Kolff was head of the department of artificial organs. In his quest to build an artificial heart, Kolff needed a mechanical or electrical pump small enough to fit in the human chest cavity but strong enough to duplicate the heart's action. Thompson Products, Inc., in Cleveland, and retired engineer S. Harry Norton, first became involved in the heart-pump project in January 1957.

Kolff thought that the fuel pump of a truck might be similar to what he wanted. He asked various motor companies to furnish him with standard pumps. One company even assigned an engineer to develop a pump design to meet Kolff's needs. However, ordinary truck pumps pump only about one liter of liquid a minute; Kolff's had to pump five liters a minute. Kolff moved both blood and a saline solution, which has characteristics similar to blood, through the pumps. Kolff learned that automotive fuel pumps worked in a way opposite to the action of the human heart.

Reversing the piston movement on the truck pump to make it work like the heart movement, Norton built several different models. One early pump was driven by electromagnets, but it was not efficient. Next they tested small electric motors to drive the pumps. One, called a pendulum heart, had a motor that swung back and forth, alternately compressing the separated right and left ventricles. Another was a roller type of pump. In that model a roller passed over the ventricle, squeezing out the blood. Experiments continued.

In 1960 Kolff described his vision of the artificial heart in the November 14 issue of *Newsweek*: "It will be a small motor-driven pump. Two wires will come out of the chest and into a portable battery. The battery will last long enough to take you from one electrical outlet to another, or to the cigarette lighter in your car."

However, the electrical motors were found to be inefficient. They were weak, heavy, and generated too much heat. Someone suggested to Kolff that he use compressed air instead of electricity. He resisted the idea since that meant the power supply would have to be outside the body. But in that year medical and industrial teams began devising artificial hearts driven by compressed air. This more efficient and powerful type of drive produced the desired result, so Kolff agreed to its use.

Medical obstacles

But even after a successful pump with external power sources was developed, many medical obstacles remained. Such obstacles included the body's nervous system, blood flow during activity, attaching the artificial heart to arteries successfully, and rejection of the strange device by the human body. The problems seemed endless.

One obstacle was solved with a human-made fabric. The challenge was to develop a pump interior that would not destroy fragile blood cells. The engineering research teams of Baylor University College of Medicine and Rice University, both in Houston, solved this problem when they discovered nylon velour. It was perfect for lining the pump. The soft, peach-fuzz material kept delicate blood cells from being bruised and ruptured.

Animals test first artificial hearts

Blood composition proved to be a problem with the plastic hearts. Blood tended to form clots on the plastic material. The clots then drifted into the bloodstream and plugged vessels in vital organs, causing experimental animals to die. By 1965 the preferred material for implantable substitute human hearts was Dacron-reinforced silicone rubber. Silicone rubber was flexible, compatible with body tissues, and easy to sterilize.

Silicone-rubber artificial hearts driven by compressed air were first tested on dogs and calves. In 1965 Dr. Kolff selected a calf to test the artificial heart for two reasons: a calf's blood clots more like a human's blood, and a calf's weight and heart volume are similar to human measurements. Connected to compressed-air lines and monitoring and control equipment, the fully conscious calf, using Dr. Kolff's replacement heart, was kept alive for thirty-one hours and showed no signs of suffering. "Long-term success in the calf is the only remaining prerequisite [requirement] for use of the artificial heart in humans," said Dr. Kolff in a June 1965 article in *Today's Health*. The permanent artificial heart was the goal, but it would not be easily accomplished. However, many other human-made devices to keep the heart functioning would be developed in the meantime.

After a decade of animal experimentation, doctors in Houston and Brooklyn, New York, implanted mechanical heart devices into humans. These were designed specifically to aid a failing left ventricle of the heart. Most heart-related deaths are due to left ventricle failure—a dysfunction of the heart's main pumping chamber. Even if death does not occur, heart attacks usually damage the left ventricle in varying degrees. Artificial ventricles were for temporary use only, until the patient's own heart could function again without assistance.

In 1963 Houston's daring surgeon Dr. Michael E. DeBakey implanted a device that took over much of the work of one patient's diseased heart for three days. A weakened left ventricle was aided by an implanted silicone-plastic, banana-shaped apparatus that was attached to an exterior air pump. Although the patient died, doctors thought this half-heart replacement could prove

The Division of Artificial Organs at Salt Lake City's University of Utah shows animal experimentation. Calves in this lab have had artificial hearts or heart boosters implanted in them.

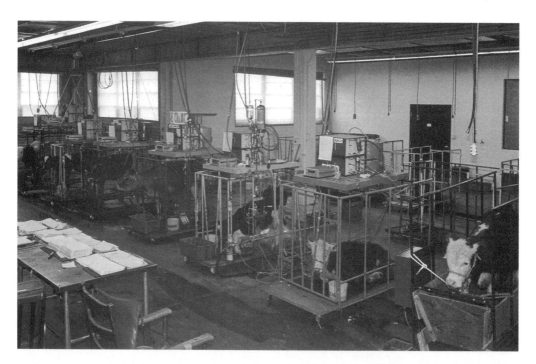

useful to other patients with diseased hearts because it gave the left ventricle a rest and allowed it to regain strength.

In 1966 in another step toward a workable mechanical heart, two dying patients received artificial heart boosters. The first patient had surgery in April 1966 at the Methodist Hospital in Houston, where Dr. DeBakey implanted a clear plastic dome heart pump about the size of a grapefruit. The dome rested on the patient's chest, with its tubes connected to his heart and to a twenty-five-pound motor beside the bed. This device kept blood pressure and circulation at normal levels while damaged areas of the heart got a chance to heal. The bypass or booster pump was not a complete artificial heart but a heart helper. The operation was technically known as a left ventricle bypass. The history-making first patient, Marcel DeRudder, lived for one hundred hours.

The second patient had surgery the following month, by a different heart surgeon, Dr. Adrian Kantrowitz, who implanted his own design of a left ventricle pump into a patient at Brooklyn's Maimonides Hospital. Unlike DeBakey's exterior

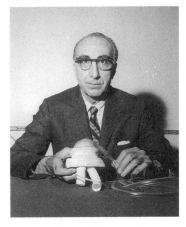

Dr. DeBakey holds a dome-shaped left ventricle pump similar to the one he implanted into a patient in 1966.

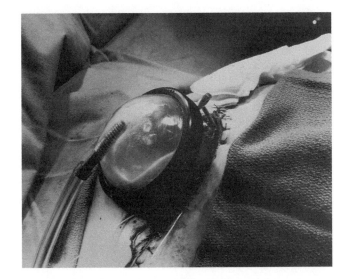

A heart booster shown resting on Marcel DeRudder's chest kept him alive for one hundred hours. The exterior tubes were connected to a twenty-five-pound motor next to his bed.

booster pump, the Kantrowitz-Avco booster (developed with the help of the Avco Corporation) was sewn permanently inside the chest cavity and attached to the aorta. The bypass shunt could be turned on and off. The patient, sixty-three-year-old Louise Ceraso, was near death from diabetes and suffered from a failing kidney, liver, and heart.

Due to badly damaged hearts, both surgeries were the patients' only chances for survival. Unfortunately, both patients died, but of causes other than pump failure.

The first patient to recover after the implantation of a partial artificial heart was Esperanza del Valle Vasquez. DeBakey installed her left ventricle bypass pump in July 1966. For ten days the pump took over as much as 60 percent of her heart's duties, giving her damaged heart time to heal.

By that time it was becoming obvious that artificial parts could help decrease the nearly one million deaths in the United States every year from heart disease. The National Heart Institute

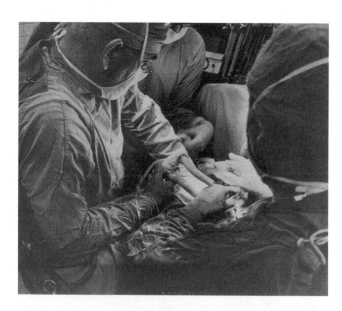

Dr. Adrian Kantrowitz implants his version of a mechanical heart booster into the chest of Louise Ceraso to assist her failing left ventricle.

(NHI) in Bethesda, Maryland, proposed a massive sixteen-billion-dollar research and development program to be conducted between 1966 and 1985. Their goal was to develop emergency, partial, and total artificial replacement devices that could be used to extend the lives of heart patients.

A total artificial heart

In April 1969 in Houston, Dr. Denton A. Cooley, who had transplanted more human hearts—eighteen—than any other surgeon, found human hearts in short supply. At that time in order to save a failing heart patient, he implanted the world's first total artificial heart as a stopgap measure while waiting for a suitable heart donor.

The patient was Haskell Karp, age forty-seven. Although Karp received an internal artificial heart, he was attached by two thin air hoses to an external power system housed in a cabinet as big as a refrigerator. The artificial heart, developed by Dr. Domingo Liotta, who had studied under both Drs. Kolff and DeBakey, beat for nearly sixty-three hours in Karp's chest. Then it was replaced by a human-donated heart. Sadly, Karp died from pneumonia and kidney failure thirty hours after the heart transplant. Karp's death immediately touched off controversy over whether the total artificial heart should have been used without further animal experimentation.

In the April 18, 1969, issue of *Time*, Cooley said, "It was an act of desperation. I was concerned of course, because this had never been done before." Karp's death prompted questions about whether the heart had undergone the required tests and scientific review before the operation. Experimental medical devices developed with federal funds require scientific review before they are used in humans. Federal guidelines state that when federal money is used any "scientific

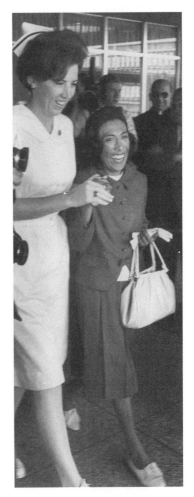

Esperanza del Valle Vasquez walks out of Houston's Methodist Hospital after undergoing surgery to receive a partial artificial heart.

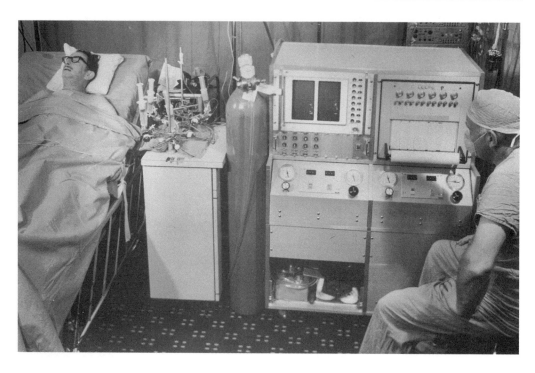

Dr. Denton Cooley monitors Haskell Karp's condition after performing the world's first total artificial heart surgery. The temporary replacement was used only for sixty-three hours until a human heart became available for transplant.

and ethical matters involved [must] be reviewed by scientists and physicians at the hospital not [by those] involved in the experiments."

Some researchers said that the heart had been developed with federal funds while Cooley contended that it had not. The *Time* reporter wrote: "As a result of the furor provoked by the Karp case and the still unresolved questions of procedure and ethics, heart surgeons are likely to be extremely hesitant before they try to duplicate Dr. Cooley's desperate act."

By 1970 the National Heart Institute had awarded some ninety million dollars in contracts to universities, hospitals, and electronic, chemical, and engineering firms in an all-out effort to perfect artificial-heart-replacement pumps, booster pumps, and heart-lung machines for open-heart surgery. By this time some twenty models of fully functioning artificial hearts had been designed with NHI support, although none of these had been tested in humans. The NHI's Artificial Heart Program had two objectives: a total mechanical heart, which completely and irrevocably replaces a person's natural one; and a booster heart, or implanted pump, temporary or permanent, to assist the patient's own heart.

The next year Dr. Adrian Kantrowitz implanted the first auxiliary, or supporting, plastic heart into the chest of Haskell Shanks. The artificial organ, a balloon pump sewn into his aorta, was placed next to Shanks's natural heart. Used as a heart-assist device, it took over about half the pumping load. Shanks was the first person to actually leave the hospital with a functioning heart-assist device. He wore a vest that contained batteries, a one-and-a-half-inch motor, and a one-inch pump that was plugged into his chest. He lived three months and three days before dying of kidney failure.

The historic Jarvik-7 model

Finally, in 1981 a total mechanical heart, the Jarvik-7, was ready for humans. It had been in development stages for eleven years. The last test subject before human testing began, a calf, had lived 268 days on a Jarvik-7 artificial heart specially adapted for use in animals.

Haskell Shanks and a nurse, in 1971, after successful heart assist surgery.

The Jarvik-7, designed by thirty-six-year-old bioengineer-physician Robert Jarvik, received approval for use in humans by the University of Utah's Institutional Review Board. Next it had to get approval from the U.S. Food and Drug Administration (FDA), which monitors clinical trials of new medical devices. On September 10, 1981, the FDA authorized the Jarvik-7 for human experimentation. The Jarvik-7 was an 8.8-ounce aluminum and plastic heart. It was slightly larger than an average heart. It had four Dacron connectors that had to be sewn onto the ends of the two

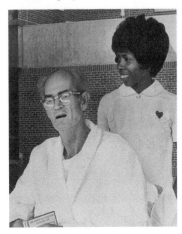

The Jarvik-7 artificial heart was designed by bioengineer-physician Robert Jarvik.

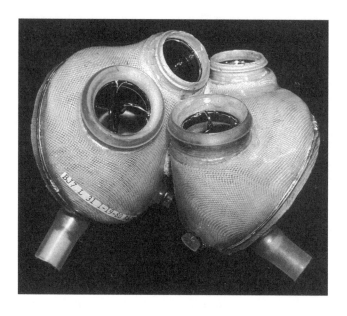

Dr. Robert Jarvik holds the Jarvik-7, the first permanent total artificial heart device approved by the U.S. Food and Drug Administration (FDA).

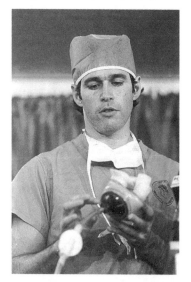

atria, the aorta, and the pulmonary artery. The hollow ventricular chambers snapped, like Tupperware, into the grooved circular connectors.

Dr. William C. DeVries, age thirty-eight, chief of cardiovascular surgery at the University of Utah Medical Center in Salt Lake City, received permission from the FDA to implant the Jarvik-7 heart as soon as a suitable patient became available. Dr. DeVries had spent three years implanting Jarvik hearts into animals and cadavers and had studied under Dr. Willem Kolff. The patient selected for surgery had to satisfy a long list of requirements including an incurable heart condition and the absence of other serious ailments.

Barney Clark, a sixty-one-year-old dentist, teetering on the edge of death, was the first to meet the rigorous criteria. He received the first permanently implanted total artificial heart on December 2, 1982. The courageous Clark knew the risk he was taking in this history-making procedure. He might die on the operating table, or he might live for an unknown time, linked by plastic tubing to the air compressor that drives the artificial heart.

This first permanent artificial-heart surgery was performed by a team of fourteen surgeons, cardiologists, nurses, and technicians and took seven and a half hours. The Jarvik-7 heart was connected to Clark's two natural atria that had been left in place. To keep the heart pumping blood, Clark was permanently tethered to 375 pounds of equipment on a cart. Because this air compressor greatly inhibited mobility, the next goal would be to design a heart that allowed a patient more independence. Still, Clark's surgery offered new hope for people with diseased hearts.

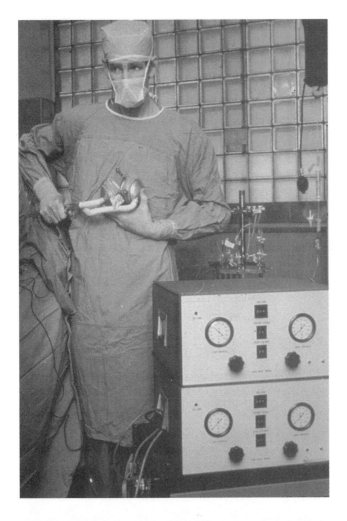

Cardiovascular surgeon William DeVries (pictured) prepares to implant the Jarvik-7 heart into patient Barney Clark.

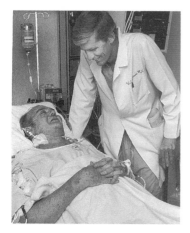

Dr. DeVries visits his famous patient Barney Clark.

Clark's courage and stamina had topped the list of reasons for his selection as a recipient. He needed both. After suffering seizures and undergoing two additional surgeries—one on a lung and one to correct a defective valve on his mechanical heart—as well as pneumonia and nosebleeds, Clark slowly improved. Although he suffered from depression, confusion, and hallucinations and even wanted to die at times, Clark stated in the March 14 and April 4, 1983, issues of *Time*: "It *is* worth it." He advised other artificial-heart candidates to go ahead with the procedure "if the alternative is they die or have it done. . . . All in all, it has been a pleasure to be able to help people. . . . If I can make a contribution, my life will count for something."

After fourteen weeks Clark was eating a varied diet, taking cautious steps with a walker, pumping a modified exercise bicycle, and talking. However, after 112 days, Clark died due to circulatory collapse and multiorgan failure—but not

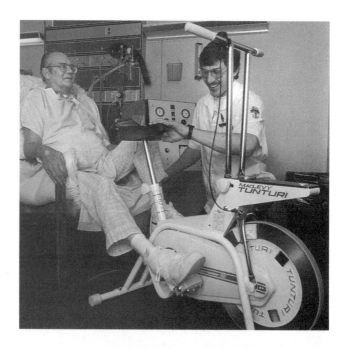

Clark begins to rebuild his strength by pedaling a specially rigged bicycle about three months after receiving his artificial heart.

due to any failure of the artificial heart, which was still pumping. Barney Clark is considered one of the great pioneers in the history of medical research.

A second human volunteer

In November 1984—almost two years after Barney Clark's implant—a second patient, fifty-two-year-old William J. Schroeder, received a revised version of the Jarvik-7 artificial heart. The original model's two-piece valves had been replaced by a stronger one-piece titanium design. This redesigned heart could be powered for two to three hours a day by a twelve-pound portable power pack the size of a camera bag, which could be worn over the shoulder. Schroeder was the first person to use the portable power pack, known as the Heimes Heart Driver unit, and developed by West German inventor Dr. Peter Heimes. At other times Schroeder was connected to a bulky 320-pound air compressor that powered his heart. Dr. DeVries, now at Humana Heart Institute, a private hospital in Louisville, Kentucky, performed the surgery.

Bionic Bill, as Schroeder was dubbed by tabloids, died on August 7, 1986, after 620 days, making him the longest surviving implant recipient at the time. The complications Schroeder suffered after receiving his artificial heart included strokes, seizures, depression, and fever and flu-like illnesses. He received blood transfusions and a variety of drugs, some experimental. Despite the rocky course, he also experienced good days that allowed him to live in an apartment near the hospital, go fishing, attend a Louisville Cardinals baseball game, and visit his hometown of Jasper, Indiana. These notable achievements provided a hopeful vision for future recipients of artificial hearts.

William Schroeder is shown waving from the porch of his Jasper, Indiana, home nine months after receiving his artificial heart.

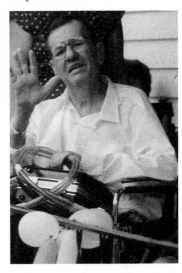

A drawing of the Jarvik-7 shows how the ventricles are stitched in place. Catheters exit through the abdominal wall and are attached to the heart driver.

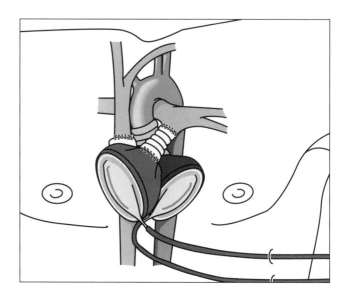

The February 1985 issue of *Life* magazine reported the following excerpts from the seventeen-page consent form that William J. Schroeder signed:

> I am fully aware of the considerable public interest anticipated in my story as a recipient of a Total Artificial Heart. . . . No representations have been made to me either that the procedure will be successful, or the length of time or the level at which the Total Artificial Heart will function. I nevertheless accept the risks of substantial and serious harm, including death, in the hope . . . that scientific information may be obtained which may be useful to others or myself. . . . [I understand that] this implantation may shorten my life and/or reduce the quality of my remaining life."

In the years following the dramatic operations performed on Barney Clark, William Schroeder, and a few others, controversy over the use of the Jarvik-7 artificial heart surfaced. Of the five people who had received the hearts, four of the five had suffered disabling strokes, and three had died. Heart specialists and others questioned whether the experiment should continue. One area of concern was cost.

Although Clark's treatment, estimated at more than $200,000, was paid for from private donations, issues related to funding the artificial-heart program brought up troubling questions. The device, operation, and hospital care would cost about $100,000 a recipient in the first year after implantation.

If the artificial heart were perfected, and the government was unwilling to pay for the operations of all who needed it—projected at sixteen thousand to sixty-six thousand heart patients each year—the device would be available only to the wealthy. It would be unfair to allow only the wealthy to benefit from the $200 million federally funded program that had developed the device. If Medicare were extended, as it had been to artificial kidney recipients, to include artificial heart patients, there would be a $5.5 billion drain on the nation's health-care system.

In addition, many experts still believed that aggressive basic research, rather than mechanical hearts, offered the best answer to cardiac disease. Some worried that federal funding of a massive artificial-heart program would mean continued neglect of research on the prevention of heart disease. In the April 4, 1983, issue of *Newsweek*, Daniel Callahan of the Institute of Society, Ethics and Life Sciences in New York said: "The artificial heart took millions to develop and will require millions more to be perfected."

The work continues

By this time, however, Utah researchers had changed their thinking on the artificial heart. They agreed that it was most useful as a bridge to transplantation—maybe for several weeks—until a human-heart donor could be located. They also agreed that research on the artificial heart should continue for several reasons. The human body

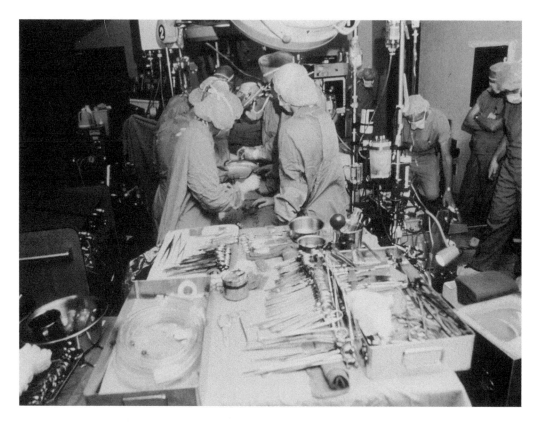

The surgical team at the University of Utah Medical Center prepares for the implantation of Clark's Jarvik-7. The high cost of developing the artificial heart has caused some experts to question whether research money would be better spent on cardiac disease prevention.

seemed to accept the plastic artificial heart, eliminating the need for the antirejection drugs required in human-heart transplants. Also, artificial hearts could be mass-produced to get around the chronic shortage of human hearts.

The April 4, 1983, issue of *Maclean's* supported this view:

> Although a conventional heart transplant from a human donor is the preferred option, there are not enough donor hearts to meet the demand. Even South African transplant pioneer Dr. Christiaan Barnard, initially skeptical of the artificial heart, reversed his stand and urged the Utah doctors last week to "go on with the work." If they succeed, Barney Clark's painful struggle and his death will not have been in vain.

By February 1987, however, the Jarvik-7 artificial heart was believed to be an unfulfilled promise. In 1988 the National Heart, Lung, and Blood Institute tried to back out of contracts that called for continued studies for a total artificial heart. They worried that scientists were still a decade or two away from solving problems with the materials, the force of the pumps, and of finding a safe miniature power source. Concerns had also been raised about the connection between the artificial heart and disabling physical problems such as anemia and strokes. Congressional pressure forced the institute to honor its contracts, but deficiencies in clinical trials led to a 1990 ban on their use even as a temporary bridge to human-heart transplants. Dr. William DeVries explains further:

> By January [1990], the FDA banned the company that manufactured the Jarvik-7 artificial heart from allowing further implantation. They felt that the company was not reporting the results accurately. Several years later the ban on the Jarvik-7 was lifted after a new company, Cardiowest, had bought the rights to begin to manufacture and study the artificial heart. To date, Jarvik-type hearts have been implanted in over 300 patients while awaiting heart transplantation.

The quest for a permanent, fully functioning artificial heart continues, however. Inventors are working on new devices for the external power tubes that would be fully implanted along with a tiny power pack in the patient's chest. The first models are expected to be ready for clinical trials around the year 2000.

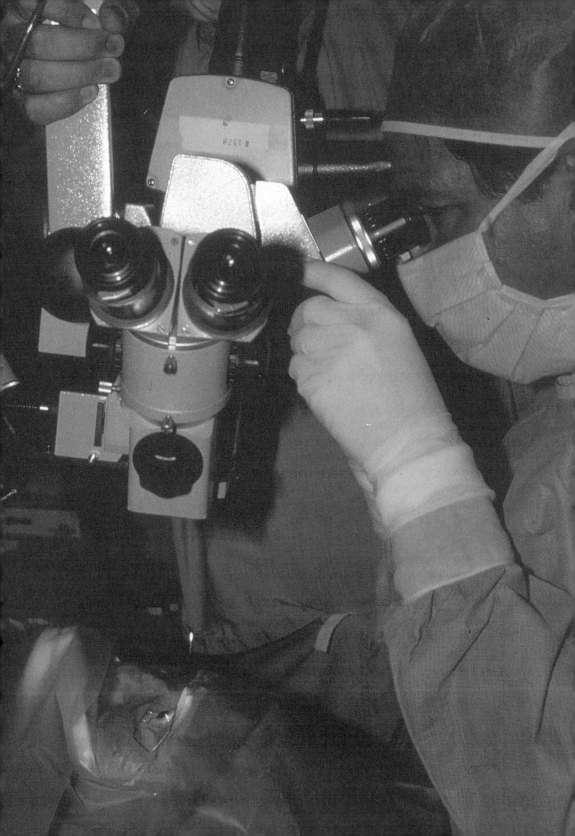

5

Artificial Sensory Organs

THE FIVE SENSORY organs form one of the most important systems of the body. People learn about the world through hearing, seeing, feeling, tasting, and smelling. Two of the body's most important senses are hearing and seeing. Both play crucial roles in communication and in the way people relate to their surroundings. Enabling deaf people to hear and blind people to see were the goals of the daring medical innovators and pioneers who first implanted artificial organs in the skull to replace faulty natural organs. But first, medical scientists needed to learn more about how the sensory organs work.

How the ear works

(Opposite page) Scientists have made remarkable progress in developing artificial sensory organs that can restore some function to damaged or diseased eyes, ears, and skin. High-powered microscopes and delicate instruments assist surgeons who perform a cataract operation to restore a patient's sight.

The development of the first artificial ear followed research into the workings of the ear and how its various parts hear sounds. By the 1950s researchers already knew that the ears funnel sound vibrations, turn them into nerve signals, and relay the signals to the hearing part of the brain. They also knew that the ear has three major parts: outer, middle, and inner. The outer ear consists of visible skin, tough tissue called cartilage, an ear canal, and a stretchy eardrum. The middle

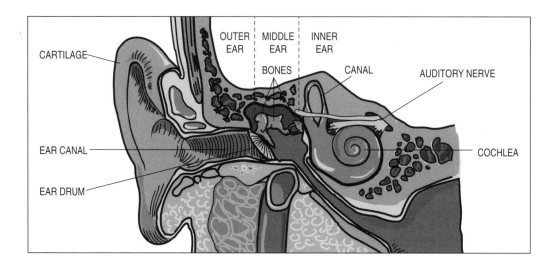

ear is an airy chamber containing three tiny bones—the hammer, anvil, and stirrup. The inner ear exists within the skull, and its parts include the semicircular canals and the spiral-shaped tube known as the cochlea.

The entire cochlea is the size of a pea, and if the spiral was unwound, it would be one and a half inches long. Inside the cochlea are more than twenty thousand microscopic hair cells that send electrical impulses from the auditory, or hearing, nerve to the brain. Over a span of twenty years, scientists learned that various locations along the cochlea are responsible for pitch, volume, texture, and quality of sound. So their work focused on the development of a cochlear implant that would allow some deaf people to hear.

The first artificial ear

Dr. William House of the House Ear Institute in California, and researchers at the 3M company of Minnesota produced the first practical cochlear implant in the 1960s. Sometimes called an artificial ear, the cochlear implant allowed patients to detect a variety of sounds. These sounds did not translate to hearing entire words, however, and patients were forced to continue using their lipreading and sign language skills. Even with its limitations, the cochlear implant was considered a breakthrough in artificial-organ technology. Its invention marked the beginning of the use of electrical stimulation inside the skull, which would eventually improve both hearing and sight. That stimulation was accomplished through the use of a tiny electrode, a wire through which an electric current passes.

Breaking the barrier of deafness

The artificial ear actually consists of two electronic assemblies: one outside the head and one surgically implanted inside the head. The external package detects sound and transmits signals to the implanted electronics. The internal package receives transmitted signals and converts them so they can stimulate the cochlea and therefore be perceived by the auditory nerve.

The external equipment includes three devices: a tiny microphone, smaller than a Chex cereal piece, usually worn behind the ear; a battery-powered processor, about the size of a pager, which can be clipped to a belt or worn in a pocket; and a transmitter about the size of a nickel, which is worn above and behind the ear. The microphone picks up sound and converts it to electrical impulses. The processor converts the electrical impulses in order to stimulate the cochlea and sends the impulses through a thin cable to the transmitter. At this point the transmitter changes the impulses to magnetic signals, which pass through the skin. The implanted equipment includes a receiver and wire electrodes. The receiver, implanted just under the skin and back-to-back with the transmitter, sends signals to the cochlea through a wire electrode. There nerve fibers are stimulated, and the brain gets the message of sound.

The 3M-House Cochlear Implant mimics the function of the hair cells, which convert sound waves to electrical impulses. The single-channel device had one electrode implanted into the cochlea. The implant is more beneficial for people who lost their hearing after they learned to speak than for people who were born deaf because the former have knowledge of sounds. Clinical trials of single-channel cochlear implants began in 1972. In the next twelve years 450 patients had the cochlear implant surgery performed at the House Ear Institute.

After the surgery these patients could recognize sounds, but they could not understand words without visual cues. Even though speech was unintelligible, the cochlear implant was an important advance. It has "broken the barrier of deafness which has plagued men, women, and children for thousands of years" said its developer, Dr. William House, in the December 10, 1984, issue of *Newsweek*. In December 1984 the Food and Drug Administration approved the electronic cochlear implant for public use. The battery-powered cochlear-implant system was the first artificial device the FDA had ever approved to replace a human sensory organ.

Multichannel implants

But for all the hope it offered, the single-channel cochlear implant still could not give the deaf the ability to distinguish words without using lipreading. Ultimate success of a cochlear implant would not be achieved until the deaf patients who received the implant could recognize words with their eyes closed. This goal, then, became one of the challenges for scientists and inventors.

What resulted was the multichannel cochlear implant. Researchers at Stanford University in California, one of several institutions developing

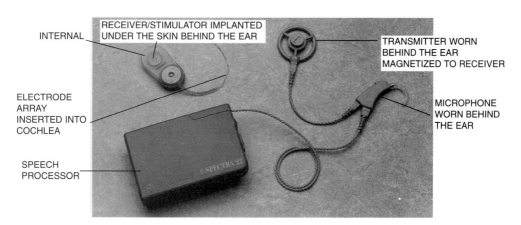

INTERNAL

RECEIVER/STIMULATOR IMPLANTED
UNDER THE SKIN BEHIND THE EAR

TRANSMITTER WORN
BEHIND THE EAR
MAGNETIZED TO RECEIVER

ELECTRODE
ARRAY
INSERTED INTO
COCHLEA

MICROPHONE
WORN BEHIND
THE EAR

SPEECH
PROCESSOR

a multichannel system, began clinical trials in 1985. Designed by Professor F. Blair Simmons, the Stanford model consisted of a bundle of eight electrodes—wires and contacts—threaded into the cochlea. By sending information through several electrodes, a multichannel implant had the ability to provide more sound cues than did a single-channel one. It stimulated more than just one spot on the cochlea. Today this device still does not allow normal hearing. Voices and words sound electronic or robotlike. However, with time and practice, wearers find that sounds and voices are more easily understood.

By 1993 there were about two hundred cochlear-implant centers across the United States. These centers have performed more than seven thousand cochlear-implant surgeries, over two thousand of them on children. Multichannel users report 30 to 95 percent speech understanding without lipreading. No one has had normal hearing completely restored by the cochlear implant, but virtually all recipients receive some measurable benefit from their implants.

Coming back to the hearing world

In May 1987, after years of living in a silent world, two Michigan girls became the first

Shown are the internal (upper left) and external components of the Nucleus 22 Channel System.

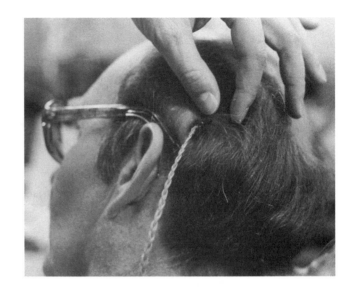

A deaf volunteer in the University of Utah's artificial hearing project is shown with a transmitter and microphone behind his ear. They are attached to a speech processor (not shown).

A man with a cochlear implant holds the speech processor which fits into his shirt pocket.

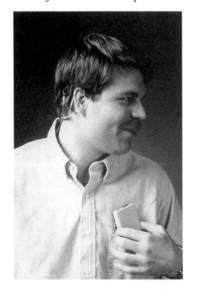

teenagers to receive the Nucleus 22 Channel Cochlear Implant. To enter the hearing world, the girls had to undergo a two-phase process. The first phase required surgery to implant a tiny audio receiver in the bone behind the ear and to insert an electrode bundle into the cochlea. Six weeks later, in the second phase, they were given the system's external parts: the microphone and the transmitter, both worn behind the ear, and the speech processor, which looks like a Walkman. The surgery changed the lives of the profoundly deaf girls. "It's like a whole new world," Brenda Jones told *Seventeen* magazine. "Every day there are new sounds. I can't wait to hear new ones, to learn more. It's great."

The second teenager, Karrie McCoy, was the center of attention at her school where other hearing-impaired students had followed Karrie's progress and filled a scrapbook with newspaper articles about her operation. "The first day back at school," Karrie said, "everyone was asking, 'Can you hear me? Can you hear me? What do I sound like?'" Even though it will take years of practice to fine-tune their understanding of sounds, these two teenagers can now enjoy being part of the hearing world.

The amount of hearing improvement realized by patients depends on their determination and the supportive help of family members. There is no doubt about the value of the cochlear implant. It can relieve social isolation and depression for profoundly deaf people. Feelings of isolation and depression are also common in people who have lost another of the five senses, the sense of sight.

Artificial eye parts

A fully functioning artificial eye is still in experimental stages, but researchers have had some success in restoring vision with the use of artificial eye parts. One eye part, the lens in the eyeball, can become cloudy. When the lens is no longer transparent, the cloudiness interferes with the passage of light rays to the retina and causes partial or near total blindness. This causes a condition known as a cataract. Cataracts are related to the aging process. Two-thirds of people over age sixty have some vision loss from cataracts. Occasionally, cataracts are caused by diabetes, injuries, and other conditions. An artificial lens implanted in the eye has been particularly successful in treating cataracts.

Cataract research got an unexpected boost in the 1940s, during World War II. European eye specialists noticed that when British airmen got pieces of plastic from exploding plane windows embedded in their eyes, the eyes did not reject the plastic. The realization that plastic could survive in the eye environment without doing harm offered new possibilities for treating eye problems.

A solution for cataracts

Ophthalmologists, doctors who specialize in eye diseases, began developing a plastic replacement

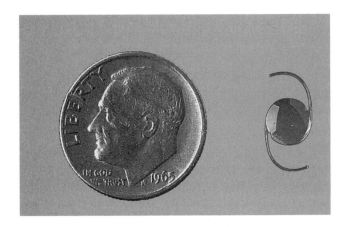

for the cloudy eye lens. The biggest challenge was to keep the lens from dropping out of position. Every design failed until the 1960s. A Dutch ophthalmologist, Dr. Cornelius D. Binkhorst, was the first to succeed by clipping the plastic lens to the iris, or colored part of the eye. This method of attachment kept the lens in place and allowed patients to see perfectly or with mildly corrective eyeglasses.

There are no proven medical ways to prevent or reverse lens clouding. Only surgical removal of a cataract and implanting a new lens restores vision. Modern cataract surgery is performed on about one million patients a year. Cataract surgery today is 97 percent successful in significantly restoring vision. A cataract is removed by using an operating microscope and delicate miniaturized instruments. The surgeon removes a tiny portion of the front capsule, or outer layer, of the lens. Through that incision the cataract is shattered into small particles with an ultrasonic device and then removed by suction. The surgery leaves the edges and back capsule of the lens in place. When the natural lens is removed, a new way to focus light must be provided.

In the past very thick eyeglasses or a contact lens had to be used. However, these were not always suitable. Nowadays a soft or hard transparent plastic lens is implanted, usually behind the iris. The tiny one-quarter-inch intraocular lens—the lens inside the eye—is supported by adjoining eye structures with a variety of springy hooks or loops and implanted permanently. The lenses are available in many designs and prescriptions, since they also correct other vision problems such as farsightedness and nearsightedness.

Successful implanting of artificial parts in ears and eyes to aid hearing and seeing encouraged researchers to study another sensory part of the body—the skin. One goal was to develop artificial skin that would save the lives of burn victims.

What does skin do?

Skin is the largest organ of the body. About the thickness of a dime, skin has two layers. The lower layer, the dermis, is spongy. It stores hair follicles, sweat glands, and nerve endings. The upper or outer layer, the epidermis, is composed mostly of scalelike cells. These are pushed upward toward the surface and are shed about every two weeks. The wonder of skin is that it is self-renewing. Some of the functions of the skin include protecting the body, regulating body temperature, perceiving touch, and keeping blood and water inside the body.

When a person is so severely burned that both layers of skin are destroyed, this is usually diagnosed as third-degree burns. Burn victims often die because they do not have skin to keep out bacteria or to retain body fluids. Of the estimated 130,000 burn victims each year in the United States, 10,000 die.

Third-degree burns are horribly painful. Wounds are covered with a variety of temporary coverings, then days or weeks later, the terrible ordeal of grafting begins. Grafting is the surgical

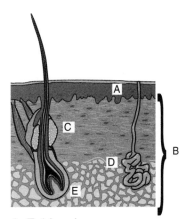

A–Epidermis
B–Dermis
C–Hairshaft
D–Sweat Gland
E–Hair Follicle

replacement of damaged skin with new skin. This process is often done in several sessions. Skin grafting is painful and usually leaves disfiguring, bumpy scars.

Developing a skin replica

When skin grafts are required, the ideal covering is the patient's own skin. The epidermal layer and part of the dermal layer can be removed from an unaffected area and placed over the wound. However, this creates two scars, and sometimes severely burned patients do not have enough good skin to cover their wounds. Skin can also be obtained from cadavers (dead bodies used for research) and pigs. Both cadaver and pig skin is temporary and will be rejected in three to twenty-five days, making it necessary to repeat the process. With these problems, the development of a synthetic skin seemed the best hope for the severely burned.

In the late 1950s Dr. John F. Burke, chief of trauma services at Boston's Massachusetts General Hospital, and one of the world's leading burn specialists, began searching for an improved kind of skin graft to help his patients. For years he and a team of doctors analyzed the chemical structure of flesh, hoping to create an artificial skin. But failure followed failure.

In December 1969 physical chemist Ioannis V. Yannas, a faculty member at Massachusetts Institute of Technology, heard of Dr. Burke's work with burn patients. Yannas had specialized in the study of collagen, the protein found in skin. They began working together. The two Boston scientists investigated a synthetic alternative to human or animal skin grafts.

Their artificial skin was like a synthetic sandwich because it had two layers, like natural skin. The dermis was made of proteins from cowhide

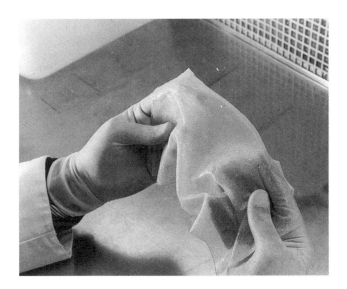

The Burke-Yannas artificial skin is about as thick as a paper towel. It is soft, pliable, and fosters the healing process much like natural skin.

and shark cartilage and was porous. The epidermis was an elastic silicone adhesive that was bonded to the cowhide-shark sheet. This artificial skin was about as thick as a paper towel. The soft and pliable sheet handled much like real skin. It was draped on burn wounds in six-by-ten-inch patches. The completed two-layer skin product could be freeze-dried and stored in sterile, closed containers.

Yannas and Burke found that the chemistry of their trial artificial skin performed as it would in a normally healing wound. That is, it healed from the outer edge toward the center, closing the wound and rejecting the covering just as a scab forms on a scrape and then falls off the fresh skin that has grown beneath it.

For the next decade the doctors experimented with guinea pigs. They removed portions of skin from anesthetized guinea pigs and covered the wounds with grafts of the experimental artificial skin. For weeks after grafting and initial healing, they watched to see how the animals would fare. The artificial skin performed as hoped, and this had been done without the use of drugs to suppress rejection. Soon they could safely experiment on a human. They were ready to tell the world.

In the May 4, 1981, issue of *Time*, the scientists shared their discovery. Dr. Burke explained the process: "The nerve fibers from below, which are still alive, grow up into the new material just like blood vessels and connective tissue. So these patients have the same sensations as with a skin graft. It isn't perfect, but it is very good."

The artificial dermis breaks down as new, natural tissue forms, and the top silicone layer acts only as a temporary protective covering. About three weeks after the artificial skin graft, the top layer is peeled away in one-inch squares and replaced by slivers of the patient's own epidermal tissue.

Promising results

In the sixteen months after the first grafts of the artificial skin on humans, results looked promising. The artificial skin appeared to maintain adequate contact between the graft and the wound, preventing air pockets that could allow infection. It seemed to be flexible enough to drape over outer elbows, under knees, and over shoulders. It resisted moisture, avoiding drying, curling, or separating. It also was biodegradable at the same rate as the new tissue growing around the wound.

Of ten severely burned patients—burned over 60 to 90 percent of their bodies—none rejected the artificial skin, none had infections, and there was little scarring. In appearance the combination of artificial skin with the patient's own tissue resembled new skin color. The patient could feel heat, cold, and touch.

Artificial skin had passed the human test, with one problem. After twenty-seven days the outer silicone layer of the skin substitute, which had acted as a temporary protective coating, had to be replaced with small pieces of epidermis from other parts of the patient's body. This skin grafting was a painful procedure. The inventors wanted to perfect a one-step process of grafting artificial skin—one in which the top layer would dissolve and form an epidermis.

Dr. Yannas explained their next goal: "We want to develop a membrane that will cover the wound and let it change over to natural skin without any more treatment or procedures. We don't want to use the patient's own skin at all."

By 1985 the Burke-Yannas artificial skin had been used on 110 patients. Artificial skin cannot save the life of every burn victim, but the vast majority of those treated with it have survived. Most survivors report near normal skin sensation without the intense, constant itch that is a common side effect of ordinary skin grafts. Despite the disfigurement and pain, most burn patients rebuild their lives, and 90 percent of patients return to work or school within six months.

Artificial sensory organs have made exceptional progress throughout the last half of the twentieth century. Cochlear implants have helped the profoundly deaf—those with no hearing—hear sounds and in some cases understand spoken words. Eyesight has been improved or restored in cataract patients by the implantation of intraocular lenses. And many burn victims have been saved and their sense of touch restored by the use of artificial skin. We move into the next century with high expectations for even more exciting inventions and development in the field of artificial organs.

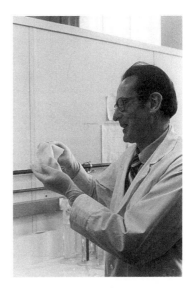

Dr. Yannas examines a sample of artificial skin, a discovery that has helped many burn victims survive.

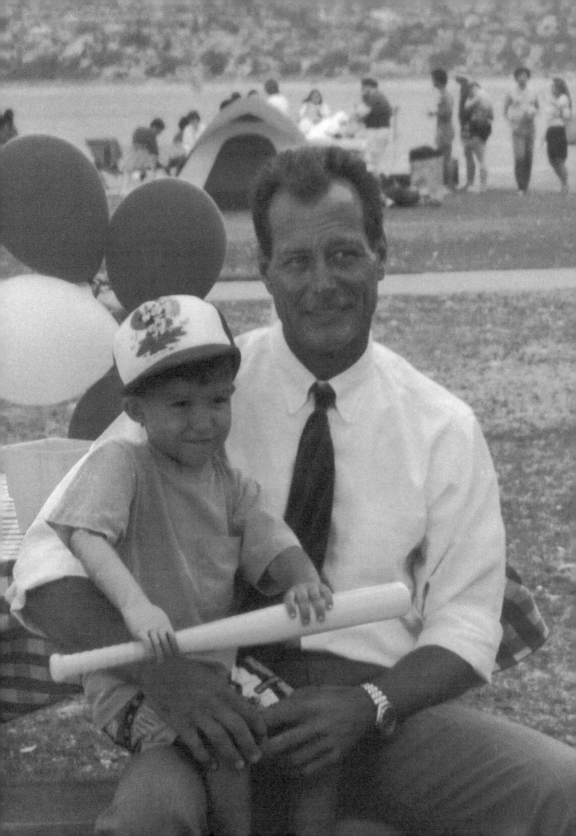

6

Merging Electronics with Artificial Organs

THE TWENTY-FIRST century is sure to bring about additional sophisticated electronic artificial organs. The understanding of how nerves and muscles are electronically stimulated by chemical response in the body was a major breakthrough. Miniature electronics are now used for artificial limbs, and rows of tiny electrodes implanted in the brain stimulate partial hearing and sight.

The idea of merging electronics with artificial organs is not new. In the late 1940s scientists explored the possibility of developing an artificial arm that used electronically stimulated muscles. But at that time electronic parts were too heavy and too large to work effectively in a human-made arm. Once electrodes became miniaturized, however, the idea of electronic artificial organs became a reality. The electronic arm is an example.

(Opposite page) Seven-year-old Shane Ynclan wears a battery-driven myoelectric arm that does not require muscle power for movement. Electrodes attached to the stump of Shane's arm detect muscle impulses, which are then transported by wire to a motor that moves his artificial arm.

Electronic arms

Unlike other artificial arms that moved by cables hooked to other parts of the body and required strenuous effort for every movement, the electronic arm requires no muscle power. All power is provided by a battery-driven electric motor mounted in the limb.

The most intriguing electronic limb is the myo-electric arm. *Myo* means muscle. *Myoelectric* refers to electrical signals in muscle fibers that trigger a contraction or movement. In an artificial arm muscle impulses are detected by electrodes placed on the remainder of the amputee's arm and passed by wires to motors that move the limbs. A myo hand looks somewhat like a human skeletal hand hooked up with wires. A skinlike glove is worn to cover the hand and about two-thirds of the prosthetic arm. The combined electronic arm and hand weighs about five pounds, only slightly less than its natural counterpart in most instances.

Utah Arm development

In 1981 at the University of Utah Center for Biomedical Design, Dr. Stephen Jacobsen and other scientists designed a revolutionary myo-electric arm that amputees could move just by thinking about it. It became known as the Utah Arm. Instead of relying on gear trains, screws, and pulleys, Jacobsen designed an artificial muscle made of flexible plastic fibers that works much like the real thing. Jacobsen had studied the role of thirty separate arm muscles involved in motion. He mapped the electrical signals sent from the muscles in an amputee's shoulder and remnant limb. These signals could be picked up by electrodes embedded in the artificial arm's socket.

Motion-control specialist Dr. Harold H. Sears explains in more detail:

> The Utah Arm has an elbow motor that can raise or lower the forearm and a motorized hand which can open and close. The amputee who is fitted with the Utah Arm must go through training and

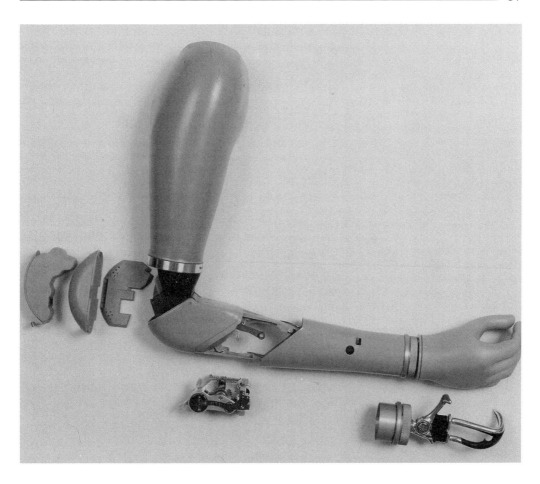

physical therapy to learn to control the muscles again, since an amputation can severely damage their muscles. Because every patient's muscle condition is different, the electronics in the arm are adjusted, or "fine-tuned," differently for each patient.

The myo arm has many advantages. It is light-weight, and the wearer is free of cables. This artificial limb also reduces the chance of curvature of the spine in children. With the old, nonpowered artificial arm, wearers had to continually twist their backs and shoulders into unnatural positions in order to activate the hook. This often resulted in deformities of the spine in children because their spines were still forming.

The Utah Arm can be used with a cosmetic hand or hook-type device. Possible motions include powered elbow bending, cable-operated holding, as well as wrist and shoulder rotation.

Unfortunately, the myoelectric arm is not satisfactory for amputees who have too few muscles left that can pick up vital signals. Other drawbacks include the high cost—up to thirty thousand dollars—size replacement every ten months for children, and the susceptibility of arm breakdown. Three years after its development, about one hundred amputees were using the myoelectric arm.

The most important factor in the success of any artificial limb, whether a new, high-tech one, or an old-fashioned one, is the attitude of the person wearing it. In the December 1988 issue of *Life* magazine, arm amputees shared their feelings about wearing prosthetic hooks and their satisfaction with the myo arm.

Reaction from electronic arm wearers

Four-year-old Alex Wright was born with his right arm missing below the elbow. At the age of ten months he was fitted for a hook with a harness attachment. This prosthetic arm required Alex to contort his shoulders to open and close the hook. The stares from people caused Alex to stop wearing his hook. Alex was next fitted with a myoelectric arm. Alex's mother says: "It's been a godsend. I wouldn't have thought appearances would be that important to a small boy, but it has made a big difference." Alex puts on his arm each morning and removes it only at bedtime. He can grip a toy golf club and swing it with gusto. He plays a child-size cello, holding the bow in his myoelectric fingers.

Eleven-year-old Glencora Hall has adjusted to her myo arm with vigorous enjoyment. Her extracurricular activities include gymnastics, drama lessons, and playing on the neighborhood softball team. Glencora says, "The best thing is when people ask me to do things without thinking, 'Oh, can she do it or should we not ask this poor disabled child?'"

The complexity of developing an electronic artificial arm was aided by the development of minute parts that can transport impulses from muscles to electrodes. Tiny electrodes have also been useful as brain implants to stimulate partial hearing and sight. Still in the experimental stages, artificial devices implanted in the brain are coming closer to restoring these senses.

Sensory implants in the brain

Daring attempts have been made to electrically stimulate the hearing nerve cells in the brain in people who have auditory nerve damage. The auditory brainstem implant (ABI) was developed to help people with neurofibromatosis type 2, a condition characterized by the growth of multiple tumors along the spinal cord and on the auditory nerves. The disorder affects one in one hundred thousand people in the United States. The tumors must be removed to prevent their growth. The tumor removal requires the severing of the auditory nerves, which in turn results in profound deafness. This condition cannot be alleviated by hearing aids or cochlear implants. The ABI offered a solution.

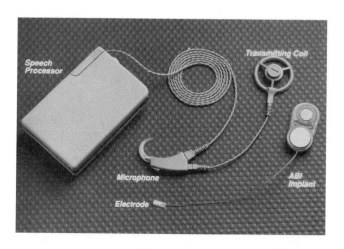

For people with auditory nerve damage the ABI is used. In this case, electrodes are implanted directly into the brain instead of the cochlea.

The ABI consists of an array, or rows, of eight electrodes inserted at the base of the brain stem beyond the auditory nerve. The electrodes allow signals to bypass the hearing nerve and to be transmitted directly to the brain. In the early 1990s the multichannel ABI was implanted into eleven patients at the House Ear Institute in Los Angeles. The ABI uses the same exterior devices—the microphone, cables, speech processor, and transmitter—as the cochlear implant. The ABI is the first commercially available brain implant that restores a sense. Preliminary results of the patients with the ABI device showed that they could hear sounds not unlike those heard by other patients with cochlear implants.

Hearing is only one sensory process accomplished through the brain. Besides sound messages, other data is sent to the brain. Eighty percent of all information received by the brain comes through the eyes.

The eye-brain connection

Many of America's six hundred thousand blind people may one day be candidates for artificial eyes—tiny video cameras mounted either on eyeglass frames or inside a glass eye. Since the 1930s researchers have known that by stimulating the visual cortex, or outer layer, of the brain, they can cause blind people to see points of light. In the 1960s several scientists investigated this phenomenon. Using blind volunteers, they placed electrodes on the surface of the visual cortex of their brains, which they stimulated with electric current. The volunteer subjects reported that they could see floating white dots.

The eyes work with the brain in processing and interpreting visual stimuli. This eye-brain connection is important to researchers who are trying to construct artificial vision systems. Vision starts at the surface of the eyeball and proceeds to the back of the brain.

In order to define the visual process in the brain, a team of University of Utah researchers directed by Dr. William H. Dobelle sought out sighted persons who were scheduled to undergo brain surgery. Between 1970 and 1974 surgeons throughout Canada and the United States were asked to notify the Dobelle team whenever a patient was diagnosed with a brain tumor in the region of the visual cortex. If a patient agreed to be part of the experiment, the team and equipment went to the patient's hospital.

They visited some sixty hospitals and did experiments on thirty-seven patients. Before the brain surgeon removed the tumor, the Dobelle research team placed electrodes against the exposed visual cortex of the patient. The brain cells were stimulated with pulses of electricity. Since the brain does not experience pain, the patient was awake during the eye experiment. During the stimulation the patient told the eye team where spots of light appeared—up, down, right, or left. This experiment showed researchers which visual brain cells were sensitive to light patterns and allowed subjects to perceive light without use of their eyes.

By 1975 the team was ready to try an electrode implant in blind volunteers. A grid of sixty-four electrodes was implanted in the visual cortex of the volunteers' brains. The volunteers were then able to describe letters and simple geometric shapes. The electronic cortical implant had wires exiting the skull that were hooked to a massive laboratory computer, which could plant visual patterns of light in the mind that the patient could "see," or perceive.

For example, a dotted Braille letter could be composed with six dots of light and allow the patient to read Braille by sight instead of touch.

Using this procedure, a blind person could read thirty characters a minute—five times faster than by using fingertips. By increasing the number of electrodes, more complicated sights, such as pictures, can be visualized by the blind patient. In the future the cortex-piercing electrode arrays could number as many as 625 to 1,024.

The artificial eye

The Dobelle team hopes to eventually create an artificial eye using a miniature video camera and a tiny computer. The camera would be fitted into a glass eye, which would be placed into a blind patient's eye socket. The glass eye would be attached to eye muscles, allowing it to move the way a normal eye moves. The camera in the glass eye would send electrical signals through wires to

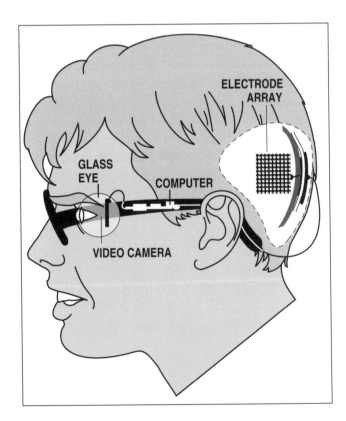

An artificial eye is still in the experimental stages. It uses a minute video camera and computer plus an electrode grid that is implanted in the brain.

a tiny computer contained in the eyeglass frame. These signals would be translated, by the computer, into information sent through wires running to electrodes on the visual cortex of the brain. Still in the early experimental stages, this artificial visual system could be a reality for commercial use in the early twenty-first century.

Dr. Richard Normann at the University of Utah describes one goal for eye researchers in *American Health* in May 1991: "We hope the blind will be able to read written text two-thirds as fast as sighted people and that they'll also be able to get around without the need for a guide dog or cane."

New ideas and research in electronics are leading researchers to a time when an artificial retina will be developed by implanting solar cell chips in the eye. In the same manner, the sense of feel or muscle movement might be restored through implanted electrodes in the area of the brain that registers the sensation of touch. This would aid stroke and paralysis victims.

A single goal

In spite of their dazzling technological successes, medical scientists say they are guided by a single goal. The January 1984 issue of *Better Homes and Gardens* quotes Dr. Willem Kolff: "The emphasis is on the restoration of happiness. We are interested in rehabilitating the whole patient, not just in replacing defective parts."

From early crude wooden devices to the development of internal artificial organs to sensory aids and electronic inventions, the lives of the disabled have been changed. Much praise and appreciation is due the many scientists and researchers who dedicate their lives to searching for ways to improve the lives of people through artificial organs.

Glossary

amputate: To cut off by surgery or by accident.

aneurysm: A blood-filled sac formed by an expanding blood vessel.

aorta: The main artery that carries blood to all bodily organs except the lungs.

atrium: An upper heart chamber that empties blood into the ventricle.

auditory: Relating to hearing organs.

auricle: The upper chamber of the heart; it receives blood through the veins then empties the blood into the lower chamber of the heart.

bioengineering: Blending engineering theories with medicine and biology.

biomaterials: Materials specifically designed by scientists to work inside the body.

cadaver: A dead body, especially one intended for dissection or research.

cardiac: Of or near the heart.

cartilage: A tough, white fibrous tissue around bone joints.

cataract: A clouding of the eye lens causing partial or total blindness.

coagulate: To form a semisolid or solid mass; to clot.

cochlea: A spiral tube of the inner ear containing nerve endings essential for hearing.

dialysis: Process of maintaining the chemical balance of the blood when the kidneys have failed. May refer to hemodialysis or peritoneal dialysis.

hemodialysis: The process of removing waste and excess water and adding chemicals to blood using an external machine.

heparin: A substance that prevents blood from clotting.

implant: An artificial material placed in a living being.

membrane: A thin sheet of natural or synthetic material through which dissolved substances can pass.

molecule: The smallest chemical unit of a material.

myoelectric: An electronic signal embedded in muscle fiber to trigger movement.

pacemaker: A device that regulates the rate of the heartbeat.

peritoneum: The membrane lining of the abdominal cavity.

polymers: A combination of molecules that form a type of plastic.

prosthesis: Any artificial part that replaces a natural body part.

pulmonary artery: An artery that carries blood between the lungs and heart.

renal: Of or near the kidneys.

septum: A strong wall dividing the left and right sides of the heart.

shunt: A device that causes fluid to change course.

socket: That part of the prosthesis that fits around the remaining limb.

suction: Drawn into by force.

synthetic: Artificial, made by humans.

transplant: Tissue or an organ transferred from one body or bodily part to another.

urea: A white crystalline or powdery compound found in urine and other body fluids.

uremia: A condition associated with the loss of kidney function and the buildup of waste products in the blood.

vascular: Tubelike vessels, such as arteries and veins, that transport blood.

ventricle: A lower heart chamber that pumps blood into the arteries.

Organizations to Contact

The following organizations can supply information about artificial organs. They will mail brochures, statistics, diagrams, and other facts. Contact them by telephone or mail.

American Amputee Foundation, Inc. (AAF)
PO Box 250218, Hillcrest Station
Little Rock, AR 72225
(501) 666-2523

AAF provides brochures and reports on the Utah Arm and partial-hand amputation and includes photographs of prosthetic arms, hands, and fingers.

House Ear Institute
2100 W. Third St., 5th Floor
Los Angeles, CA 90057
(213) 483-4431

This institute is dedicated to improving the lives of all who suffer hearing loss or balance disorders. Through research presentations and professional education and training, they share knowledge with the world. Newsletters, brochures, and reports on the cochlear implant and the auditory brainstem implant, as well as personal stories, are available.

Krames Communications
1100 Grundy Ln.
San Bruno, CA 94066-3030
(800) 333-3032

This company provides a free patient education catalog of resources on health issues. Both booklets and videos are available for purchase. Some of the topics include: feet and ankles; hands and wrists; heads, necks, and shoulders; hips; knees; surgery and physical therapy on bones; vein and artery problems; heart attacks; and eye problems. They also have booklets in Spanish.

Motion Control
1290 W. 2320 S., Suite A
Salt Lake City, UT 84119
(800) 621-3347

A division of IOMED, Inc., this company provides literature on the myoelectric hand, the Utah Arm, signal sensors, and insurance funding of the Utah Arm prosthesis.

National Kidney Foundation (NKF)
30 E. 33rd St., 11th Floor
New York, NY 10016
(800) 622-9010

Supports research, patient services, education, and community service. Branches nationwide conduct programs and services for patients and their families. The organization publishes numerous magazines and newsletters. Also available is the book *When Your Kidneys Fail*, which covers such topics as kidney function, methods of treatment, diet, and medication.

Suggestions for Further Reading

Thomas G. Aylesworth, *The Search for Life.* New York: Rand McNally, 1975.

Jacqueline Dineen, *The Five Senses.* Englewood Cliffs, NJ: Silver Burdett, 1988.

Margery Facklam and Howard Facklam, *Spare Parts for People.* San Diego: Harcourt Brace Jovanovich, 1987.

Peter Limburg, *The Story of Your Heart.* New York: Coward, McCann & Geoghegan, 1979.

Thomas H. Metos, *Artificial Humans.* New York: Julian Messner, 1985.

William A. Nolen, M.D., *Spare Parts for the Human Body.* New York: Random House, 1971.

Steve Parker, *The Ear and Hearing.* New York: Franklin Watts, 1989.

———, *The Eye and Seeing.* New York: Franklin Watts, 1989.

———, *The Heart and Blood.* New York: Franklin Watts, 1989.

Gloria Skurzynski, *Bionic Parts for People.* New York: Four Winds Press, 1978.

Alvin Silverstein and Virginia B. Silverstein, *The Sense Organs.* Englewood Cliffs, NJ: Prentice-Hall, 1971.

Barbara Taylor, *Living with Deafness.* New York: Franklin Watts, 1989.

Works Consulted

Books

Janice M. Cauwels, *The Body Shop—Bionic Revolutions in Medicine.* St. Louis: C.V. Mosby, 1986.

Donald Clark, ed., *How It Works, The Illustrated Encyclopedia of Science and Technology.* New York: Marshall Cavendish, 1978.

John G. Deaton, M.D., *New Parts for Old.* Palisade, NJ: Franklin Publishing Company, 1974.

Mickie Hall Faris, *When Your Kidneys Fail.* Los Angeles: National Kidney Foundation of Southern California, 1994.

Arthur S. Freese, *The Bionic People Are Here.* New York: McGraw-Hill, 1979.

W. J. Kolff, M.D., *New Ways of Treating Uraemia.* London, England: J. and A. Churchill, 1947.

Thomas H. Metos, *Artificial Humans.* New York: J. Messner, 1985.

George M. Pantalos, "The Future of Artificial Hearts" and "A Selected History of Mechanical Circulatory Support," in Terry Lewis, ed., *Mechanical Circulatory Support.* Sevenoaks, England: Edward Arnold Publishers. To be published.

Periodicals

Jerry Adler, "I Have Him Back Again," *Newsweek,* December 10, 1984.

Shana Alexander, "They Decide Who Lives, Who Dies," *Life,* November 9, 1962.

Alan Anderson Jr., "Dialysis or Death," *The New York Times Magazine,* March 7, 1976.

Joan Arehart-Treichel, "An Artificial Heart in Search of a Patient," *Science News,* March 7, 1981.

M. D. Bellomy, "Spare Parts for Human Hearts," *The American Mercury,* May 1960.

S. I. Benowitz, "New Life for the Artificial Heart," *Science News,* December 1, 1984.

Theodore Berland, "More Spare Parts for Humans," *Today's Health,* July 1966.

Barton J. Bernstein, "The Artificial Heart—Is It a Boon or a High-Tech Fix?" *The Nation,* January 22, 1983.

Shannon Brownlee, "Refurbishing the Body," *U.S. News & World Report,* November 12, 1990.

Business Week, "Artificial Hearts Begin to Beat," October 21, 1972.

Business Week, "Do-It-Yourself for Kidney Patients," February 4, 1967.

Business Week, "The Hunt for a Mechanical Heart," May 28, 1966.

Business Week, "Medicine and Industry Team-Up: Promises an Artificial Heart," May 17, 1958.

Malcolm N. Carter, "The Business Behind Barney Clark's Heart," *Money,* April 1983.

Laurence Cherry, "Artificial Skin: From Concept to Creation," *Reader's Digest,* September 1983.

Matt Clark, "An Incredible Affair of the Heart," *Newsweek,* December 13, 1982.

———, "New Substitutes for Skin," *Newsweek,* October 19, 1981.

———, "Stiffer Rules for the Heart," *Newsweek,* December 30, 1985.

———, "Taking Heart from Dr. Clark," *Newsweek,* February 28, 1983.

Noel L. Cohen and Michael L. Gordon, "Cochlear Implants: Basics, History, and Future Possibilities," *SHHH Journal,* January/February 1994.

Barbara J. Culliton, "Politics of the Heart," *Science,* July 15, 1988.

R. M. Cunningham Jr., "We Are Not Cripples," *Hygeia,* July 1941.

Ron Davids, "Man Made Hearts: Will They Supersede Transplants?" *Science Digest,* April 1972.

Paul F. Ellis, "'Iron Heart' Pinch-Hits for Real One," *Popular Science,* February 1951.

Robert A. Fuller and Jonathan J. Rosen, "Materials for Medicine," *Scientific American,* October 1986.

Lianne Hart, "Lives That Are Whole," *Life,* December 1988.

Larry Husten, "The Beat Goes On," *Discover,* March 1991.

Robert K. Jarvik, "The Total Artificial Heart," *Scientific American,* January 1981.

Dan Kaercher, "Amazing Advances in Medical Technology," *Better Homes and Gardens,* January 1984.

Laura Kaufman, "Eye for an Eye," *American Health,* May 1991.

T. Kleist, "Schroeder's Struggle Lasts 620 Days," *Science News,* August 16, 1986.

Jeffrey Kluger, "2001 Medicine: Rebuilding the Body, Part by Part," *Discover,* November 1988.

W. J. Kolff, "Artificial Organs — Forty Years and Beyond," *Transactions of the American Society for Artificial Internal Organs* (vol. 29, no. 789), 1983.

Willem J. Kolff, "An Artificial Heart Inside the Body," *Scientific American,* November 1965.

Alex Kucherov, "More Spare Parts for the Human Body," *U.S. News & World Report,* December 28, 1981/January 4, 1982.

Kristin Leutwyler, "Prosthetic Vision," *Scientific American,* March 1994.

Life, "Artificial Kidney," April 28, 1947.

Life, "Foot-Controlled Arm," August 7, 1950.

Life, "Rebuilt People," September 24, 1965.

Life, "Spare Parts Bank," February 17, 1958.

The Literary Digest, "'Practicable' Wooden Arms," July 31, 1915.

William D. Marbach, "Building the Bionic Man," *Newsweek,* July 12, 1982.

Eliot Marshall, "Rendezvous with a Machine," *The New Republic,* March 19, 1977.

Frank W. Martin, "Utah Surgeon William DeVries Seeks a Patient Who Could Live with a Man-Made Heart," *People,* July 19, 1982.

Mike May, "The Electric Eye," *Popular Science,* August 1993.

Charles C. McGonegal, "How I Get Along Without Hands," *Saturday Evening Post,* November 25, 1944.

John P. Merrill, "The Artificial Kidney," *Scientific American,* July 1961.

Curtis Mitchell, "Engineering the New Mechanical Heart," *Popular Science,* March 1970.

Newsweek, "The Artificial Heart," November 14, 1960.

Newsweek, "A Boost in Time," February 7, 1966.

Newsweek, "The Brooklyn Booster," June 6, 1966.

Newsweek, "An Electronic Ear to Help the Deaf Hear," December 10, 1984.

Newsweek, "Have a Heart," June 23, 1969.

Newsweek, "Heart-Lung Machine," August 8, 1949.

Newsweek, "Help for Failing Hearts," May 30, 1966.

Newsweek, "Machine of Life," July 25, 1966.

Newsweek, "The Plastic Heart," May 2, 1966.

Newsweek, "Too Much, Too Fast?" April 21, 1969.

Newsweek, "Who Is Worth Saving?" June 11, 1962.

Richard Alan Normann, "Towards an Artificial Eye," Research to Prevent Blindness Science Writers Seminar, University of Utah School of Medicine, Salt Lake City, Utah.

Pat Ohlendorf, "Lessons from the Heart," *Maclean's,* May 9, 1983.

———, "The Life Machine," *Maclean's,* December 10, 1984.

———, "Sound Device for the Deaf," *Maclean's,* May 7, 1984.

I. Peterson, "Implanting an Electronic Earful," *Science News,* November 27, 1982.

Maya Pines, "Modern Bioengineers Reinvent Human Anatomy with Spare Parts," *Smithsonian,* November 1978.

Popular Mechanics, "Body's Own Filter Material Replaces Kidneys," September 1982.

Popular Science, "Machine Cleans Blood While You Wait," January 1951.

Tom Rademacher, "The Sound of a Miracle," *Seventeen,* May 1987.

Jeanne Reinert, "Outlook for the Artificial Heart," *Science Digest,* July 1966.

John Rennie, "Who Is Normal?" *Scientific American,* August 1993.

Jhan Robbins and June Robbins, "The Rest Are Simply Left to Die," *Redbook,* November 1967.

Donald Robinson, "Who Shall Be Permitted to Live?" *50 Plus,* June 1981.

Peter F. Salisbury, "Artificial Internal Organs," *Scientific American,* August 1954.

Terri Schultz, "Advancing Technology Plus Blind Luck Equals Hope for Victor Riesel," *Today's Health,* April 1974.

Cindy Schweich, "Medical Miracles," *Redbook,* May 1991.

Science Digest, "First Artificial Heart Survivor," November 1966.

Science Digest, "The High Price of Kidney Disease," March 1972.

Science News, "Artificial Heart: The Debate Goes On," February 22, 1986.

Science News, "Cheap Kidney Developed," October 8, 1966.

Science News, "Implanting a Stopgap Heart," April 19, 1969.

Science News, "Skin for the Wounds of Burns," January 3, 1981.

Science News Letter, "Artificial Heart Valves Give Life to Patients," November 20, 1965.

Science News Letter, "Artificial Kidney Removes Poisons from Bloodstream," May 10, 1947.

Science News Letter, "Best Heart Valves Sought," January 15, 1966.

Science News Letter, "Mechanical Kidney," July 22, 1950.

Science News Letter, "Surgeons See Heart Valve," June 20, 1953.

Scientific American, "Reconstructing the War's Maimed," May 18, 1918.

Scientific American, "Tuning a Deaf Ear," November 1984.

Belding Scribner, M.D., "An Action Plan to Help Kidney Patients," *Today's Health,* December 1972.

Arthur J. Snider, "The Artificial Eye That Sees," *Science Digest,* December 1964.

Steven M. Spencer, "Artificial Arteries Can Save Your Life," *The Saturday Evening Post,* November 2, 1957.

———, "Making a Heartbeat Behave," *The Saturday Evening Post,* March 4, 1961.

Reader's Digest, "Plastic Parts for the Human Body," May 1965.

Time, "An Act of Desperation," April 18, 1969.

Time, "An Artificial Heart," April 11, 1969.

Time, "The Body May Be Best," December 18, 1978.

Time, "Five Million Beats and Counting," January 17, 1983.

Time, "Half-Heart Replacement," November 8, 1963.

Time, "Making Skin from Sharks," May 4, 1981.

Time, "Missing a Beat in Washington," April 6, 1981.

Time, "Peg Legs," October 18, 1937.

Today's Health, "AMA Honors Engineer for His Heart Valve Invention," January 1964.

Today's Health, "Auxiliary Ventricle Proposed as Aid to Ailing Hearts," February 1966.

Today's Health, "He Washes His Own Blood, Twice a Week," July 1968.

Today's Health, "How an Artificial Kidney Works," June 1961.

Today's Health, "Kidney Dialysis," January 1971.

Today's Health, "New Hearts for Old," June 1965.

J. A. Treichel, "Artificial Heart Makes Medical History," *Science News,* December 11, 1982.

U.S. News & World Report, "Man-Made Parts for the Body—Bright Future?" April 21, 1969.

U.S. News & World Report, "Step Toward a 'Mechanical Heart,'" May 2, 1966.

USA Today, "Helping Patients Live More Normal Lives," June 1982.

USA Today, "Implanted Device Fights Deafness," February 1985.

USA Today, "Turning a Deaf Ear to Helpful Implants," February 1992.

Loudon Wainwright, "A Man and His Total Artificial Heart," *Life,* February 1985.

Claudia Wallis, "Death of a Gallant Pioneer," *Time,* April 4, 1983.

————, "Feeling Much Better, Thank You," *Time,* March 14, 1983.

Joseph D. Wassersug, M.D., "Spark Plug for Ailing Hearts," *Science Digest,* November 1953.

Jennifer Westaway, "Newscience/Innovations," *Science Digest,* August 1984.

The World's Work, "Man and His Machines," June 1918.

Carl Zimmer, "Making Senses," *Discover,* June 1993.

Index

About the Author

Judith Janda Presnall was born in Milwaukee, Wisconsin, and spent her childhood there. She has a bachelor's degree in education from the University of Wisconsin, Whitewater, and taught business classes in high schools and colleges for twenty years. She began her writing career in 1985, focusing on juvenile nonfiction. Her published books include: *Animals That Glow*, awarded Outstanding Science Book for Children by the National Science Teachers Association—Children's Book Council; *The Importance of Rachel Carson*; and *Animal Skeletons*. Presnall has received awards for her writing from the Society of Children's Book Writers and Illustrators and the California Writers Club. She lives in Reseda, California, with her husband, Lance, and two cats, Penelope and Ashes. They have two grown children, Kaye and Kory.

Picture Credits

Cover photo: © Jim Olive/Peter Arnold, Inc.
Courtesy of Alcon Laboratories, Inc., 78
AP/Wide World, 40, 57 (top), 62 (bottom)
Archive Photos, 15, 42, 44
© 1994 Baxter Healthcare Corp., 24
The Bettmann Archive, 12, 16
© B.S.I.P./Custom Medical Stock, 38
The Cochlear Corporation, 75, 76 (bottom), 89
© 1993 Dan Habib/Impact Visuals, 8
© 1992 Michael McCray/Custom Medical Stock, 70
MIT New Office, 81, 83
Benjamin Montag, 92
© Hank Morgan/Photo Researchers, Inc., 10
Motion Control, A Division of IOMED, Inc., 87
National Library of Medicine, 14
RGP Prosthetic Research Center, San Diego, 84
Trinidad Tabadero, 36
TechPool, 33, 52, 66, 72, 79
University of Utah, 28, 30, 35, 50, 56, 62 (top), 63, 64 (top), 68, 76 (top)
University of Utah/Brad Nelson, 64 (bottom)
UPI/Bettmann, 18, 20, 21, 22, 47, 48, 57 (bottom), 58, 59, 60, 61, 65